Affiliation Options *for* Physicians

Current and Future Strategies

Max Reiboldt, CPA
COKER GROUP

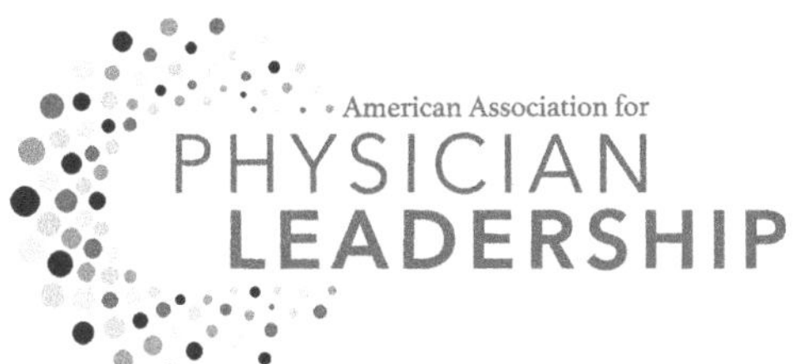

978-0-9848310-9-8 Print
978-0-9848311-0-4 eBook
Published by **American Association for Physician Leadership, Inc.**
PO Box 96503 | BMB 97493 | Washington, DC 20090-6503

Website: www.physicianleaders.org

13 8 7 6 5 4 3 2 1

Copyedited, typeset, indexed, and printed in the United States of America

PUBLISHER
Nancy Collins

EDITORIAL ASSISTANT
Jennifer Weiss

DESIGN & LAYOUT
Carter Publishing Studio

COPYEDITOR
Pat George

Table of Contents

Acknowledgments

The material in this book represents the perspectives of many contributors based on their years of working in the healthcare industry with healthcare clients. Beyond the author-contributors of Coker Group, we express special appreciation to Thomas D. Anthony, J.D., Esq., (Frost Brown Todd) for his knowledge of healthcare law. Tom is the former team leader of FBT's Health Care Innovation team. He has been honored as Best Lawyer of the Year by *The Best Lawyers in America*© 2020 for the past 10 years. *Chambers and Partners*®, a publication ranking attorneys and their practices based on peer and client review, recognized Tom in the 2019 edition of *Chambers USA*®.

We continue to enjoy working with Nancy Collins, publisher, and Jennifer Weiss, editorial assistant, and we value the confidence they share in the knowledge that Coker Group maintains. Thank you for a long and pleasant professional relationship.

Kay B. Stanley, F.A.C.M.P.E., Editor

About the Authors

Max Reiboldt, CPA, is the president/CEO of Coker Group. He has experienced first-hand the ongoing changes of healthcare providers, which uniquely equips him to handle strategic, tactical, financial, and management issues that health systems and physicians face in today's evolving marketplace.

Max understands the nuances of the healthcare industry, especially in such a dynamic age. He understands how healthcare organizations need to maintain viability in a highly competitive market. His position of having "experienced everything" in the healthcare industry equips him to provide pertinent counsel to clients. Whether a transitional provider or a more trailblazing healthcare entity, he is uniquely qualified to work with these organizations to provide sound solutions to every day and long-range challenges.

As president/CEO, Max oversees Coker Group's services and its general operations. He has a passion for working with clients and organizations of all sizes and engages in consulting projects nationwide.

A graduate of Harding University, he is a licensed certified public accountant in Georgia and Louisiana, and a member of the American Institute of Certified Public Accountants, Georgia Society of CPAs, Healthcare Financial Management Association, and American Society of Appraisers. He is also a member of the American College of Healthcare Executives. Contact Max at mreiboldt@cokergroup.com.

Thomas D. Anthony, J.D., Esq., an attorney with Frost Brown Todd, provides advice on Stark, Anti-Kickback, and all other healthcare regulatory matters. He is counsel to hospitals regarding clinically integrated networks, medical staff bylaws, physician relations, acquisition of medical groups, corporate governance, acquisitions of outpatient and ancillary facilities, strategic alliances and joint ventures, the establishment of provider-based facilities, executive employment agreements, Medicare compliance, contracting, and employment matters. He also represents several senior living facility owners and operators in mergers/acquisitions, regulatory, patient rights, and financings. Contact Tom at 513.651.6191.

Andrew Cadger is a senior associate for Coker Group's finance, operations, and strategy division. He focuses on fair market opinions, compensation model development, financial analyses, and hospital/physician alignment transactions. Andrew also works with Coker's hospital operations and strategic services team on physicians' community needs assessments and medical staff development plans. Contact Andrew at acadger@cokergroup.com.

Justin Chamblee, CPA, is a senior vice president and director of operations at Coker Group. As an executive healthcare consultant and certified public accountant, he provides strategic and financial counsel to healthcare organizations, physician practices, and healthcare attorneys throughout the country, dealing primarily with physician compensation and hospital-physician transactions. He assists healthcare organizations as they restructure their compensation arrangements to ensure they are consistent with the market on a macro and micro basis. Justin's work also includes compensation valuation, helping healthcare organizations ensure that their financial arrangements comply with the requirements of fair market value and commercial reasonableness. His work involves basic hospital-physician arrangements, such as call pay and medical directorships, to more complex agreements such as the distribution of funds from ACO/CINs and other novel value-based structures. Other areas of expertise include contract negotiations, sale/acquisition negotiations, strategic planning, and other areas of finance. Contact Justin at jchamblee@cokergroup.com.

Aimee Greeter is a senior vice president at Coker Group with specialized expertise in alignment, accountable care responsiveness, hospital service line development, clinical integration initiatives, strategic planning, executive compensation, mergers and collaborations, operational issues, and financial management. She works with nonprofit and for-profit hospitals and health systems of all sizes and larger single- and multi-specialty physician practices to achieve their strategic and tactical goals. Contact Aimee at agreeter@cokergroup.com.

Taylor Cowart is a senior associate with Coker's financial and hospital operations services division. She works predominantly in the financial and alignment services section, providing clients with consultative assistance for alignment and integration, financial analyses, and service line development. Taylor also works with accountable care era response and preparation, helping clients respond to value-based reimbursement changes and developing population health management strategies. She has extensive experience in healthcare consulting, particularly in the hospital administration arena, such as credentialing and privileging management. Contact Taylor at tcowart@cokergroup.com.

Matthew Jensen is a senior manager at Coker Group. He has more than a decade of consulting experience and is a leader in the business valuation and physician compensation valuation practice. Matthew focuses on developing valuation opinions of provider compensation agreements, healthcare-related businesses, intangible assets, and co-management arrangements. He strives to help healthcare organizations minimize risk and ensure that financial arrangements meet the complex requirements related to fair market value and commercial reasonableness opinions. Contact Matthew at mjenson@cokergroup.com.

Alex Kirkland is a vice president at Coker Group. He has more than 10 years of healthcare experience from a financial and operational background with an emphasis on physician compensation, reimbursement models, and population health. With Coker, he focuses primarily on physician alignment transactions, compensation trends, and payer reimbursement strategies.

Ellis M. "Mac" Knight, MD, formerly served as senior vice president and chief medical officer of Coker Group overseeing Coker Group's ValuePath services, designed to smooth healthcare organizations' transition from a volume-based to a value-based business model. He also directed revenue and quality integrity (RQI) services, which offer expert services around coding, compliance, and clinical documentation to healthcare organizations of all types. As chief medical officer, Dr. Knight worked on a variety of projects where his clinical background and knowledge of clinical operations brought additional value to the client. He has expertise in population health management, clinical care process design, cost accounting, clinical integration, and clinical documentation/coding improvement. He is familiar with the management and operations of rural hospitals, community hospitals, public hospitals, large health systems (to include academic medical centers), and physician practices of all types and specialties.

Christopher Kunney formerly served as senior vice president of healthcare information technology for Coker Group. He worked with hospitals, health systems, accountable care organizations, clinically integrated networks, ancillary service providers, and physician-owned entities to provide guidance and insights specific to emerging healthcare technology offerings, compliance-related issues, and technology adoption.

Erica Lindquist is a senior associate for Coker Group's finance operations and strategy division. She engages in consulting projects with physicians and health systems nationwide, providing consulting services on compensation review and model development, financial analyses, fair market value opinions, tangible asset valuations, and hospital-physician alignment transactions. Erica also assists in presentation research and development for Coker's numerous speaking engagements, as well as contributions to various healthcare magazine articles, white papers, and books. Contact Erica at elindguist@cokergroup.com.

Mark Reiboldt is senior vice president and director of strategy at the Coker Group, where he specializes in financial and transaction advisory for hospitals, medical groups, and other healthcare organizations. These transactions include mergers and acquisitions, divestitures, equity purchases, physician-alignment deals, and joint ventures. Mark's advisory services often entail acquisition/investment due diligence, valuation services, transaction management, buyside representation, strategic alternatives processes, and post-merger integration. In his role as director of strategy, he serves on the executive leadership team and works with the firm's senior management on various strategic projects. He also serves as a board member and secretary of the Coker Foundation, the firm's nonprofit charity organization. Contact Mark at markreiboldt@cokergroup.com.

Richard Romero is a senior vice president at Coker Group. His primary focus is valuation of businesses and financial arrangements, litigation support, and regulatory compliance. Additionally, he has expertise in strategic and operational consulting, bankruptcy and turnaround, expert witness services, and employment-related matters for physicians and physician practices, independent practice associations, hospitals, specialty hospitals, joint ventures, managed-care organizations, billing companies, long-term care entities, governmental entities, and research agreements. Richard has more than 20 years of experience with regulatory compliance, valuation, and litigation support. Contact Richard at rromero@cokergroup.com.

Andy Sobczyk is a manager for Coker Group's physician services and finance, operations, and strategy divisions. He partners with clients in the ambulatory enterprise to deliver value in the areas of operational efficiency, organizational structure, physician alignment strategy, financial stability, revenue cycle management, and leadership coaching and development. He also supports compensation valuation work, compensation plan redesign, and strategic business planning. Andy's previous experience includes working as a physician enterprise executive leader and a management consultant. He has a passion for collaborating with healthcare leadership, providers, and staff to identify improvement opportunities and convert strategy into meaningful action and results. Contact Andy at asobcyk@cokergroup.com.

David Walline is a senior manager in Coker Group's finance, operations, and strategy group, with a specific focus on business valuation. His business valuation career spans more than a decade, with the past eight years dedicated to the valuation of entities within the healthcare industry. David has performed hundreds of valuations on healthcare businesses, with experience working with healthcare organizations, attorneys, administrators, providers, developers, consultants, and private equity groups in connection with a broad spectrum of transactions in the healthcare industry. Contact David at dwalline@cokergroup.com.

Preface

The various options available for the affiliation of physicians can be overwhelming to potential participants, especially to those who are less familiar with the business aspects of healthcare management. Physicians, providers, administrators, and leaders across the healthcare spectrum are bombarded with possibilities for transactions. This book presents and describes the current and anticipated arrangements that offer physicians potential strategies in navigating the healthcare landscape. The best decisions can be made only with a foundational knowledge base.

Chapter One provides an overview of physician affiliation transactions with a 20-year review. The history encompasses all types of affiliations, including physician-to-physician, private group to private group, private group to hospital-health systems, private group to private equity/outside investors, and more.

Chapter Two offers an in-depth study of the financial terms and structures of the physician affiliation models that have evolved during the past 20 years.

Chapter Three details the reasons for affiliation as substantiated and supported repeatedly, especially relative to current strategies.

Chapter Four introduces current models and serves as the foundation for the subsequent chapters, which examine each model individually.

Chapter Five considers physician employment, which is the most traditional and historically based model. Considerations include practitioners in private practice and health systems, with key terms and conditions, compensation structures, and more.

Chapter Six addresses professional services agreements (PSA). PSAs are common and will continue to challenge the status of the employment model.

Chapter Seven explores joint-equity opportunities for both ancillary services and practice initiatives. This chapter focuses on equity-type structures and addresses future opportunities where physicians, hospitals, and private investors may partner.

Chapter Eight lays out the fastest-growing affiliation model between private and equity investors and physicians; *private equity transactions.* Emphasis is on the current and anticipated structures, terms, and conditions of these affiliations.

Chapter Nine considers private equity-like transactions, which is a newer concept. This model usually involves a physician (specialty) group and a health system, and it mirrors many of the features of private equity transactions.

Chapter Ten looks at clinical co-management alignment. Though it is not a standalone affiliation model, co-management is a part of other affiliation transactions, such as PSAs and employment. This chapter considers how it may apply going forward.

Chapter Eleven includes a review of several limited affiliation models, such as medical directorships, recruitment support, and others. Though these affiliations are waning, they remain popular and are worth addressing.

Chapter Twelve discusses clinically integrated networks (CINs) and value-based reimbursement (VBR) structures as a part of the transition from fee-for-service (or volume) to fee-for-value.

Chapter Thirteen addresses private groups merging in both single and multi-specialty settings, which are popular and will continue to be in the future.

Chapter Fourteen examines the role IT plays in sound decision making when healthcare entities merge. It speaks to the need for both the pre- and post-due diligence workaround information technology. Proper planning will enable both the buyer and seller to enter these transactions with full transparency and understanding of risk, including any lurking pre-existing cybersecurity threats. Discussion includes data migrations, system conversion, data archiving, application retirement, early termination, A/R burndown, reassignment of vendor contracts and support agreements, and critical success factors for achieving full IT integration.

Chapter Fifteen is devoted to various legal and regulatory compliance considerations that must be included when considering different affiliation models of the future.

Chapter Sixteen discusses options for capital procurement. While funding is primarily the purchaser's responsibility, the decisions about the options depend on the preferences of both parties. Some transactions involve minor up-front funding; others entail the exchange of substantial monies at closing. This chapter addresses the sources of financing and capitalization of the transactions of affiliation.

Chapter Seventeen is devoted to the mechanics of putting together and ultimately closing affiliation models. The process can be slow and tedious, stressing the need for engaging transaction advisory services.

Chapter Eighteen presents conclusions and provides an overview of affiliation models and structures for the future.

Chapter Nineteen wraps up the book chapters with an additional assessment of where we are as the COVID-19 pandemic has turned our country and our planet upside down. This upheaval applies to all aspects of clinical care, including the alternatives for affiliation.

The purpose of this book is to lay a strong foundation for making sound decisions about the numerous available affiliation options for physicians. The intent is to prepare the reader for the current and future healthcare practice environment. Contact Coker Group at www.cokergroup.com for more information and assistance.

CHAPTER 1

Overview of Physician Affiliation Options—50 Years of History

Through the years, the presence of physicians, hospitals, and other healthcare investors or partners has increased the complexity of the healthcare delivery system to what it is today. Though not entirely extinct, single-ownership physician practices, small locally owned hospitals, and other private healthcare entities are rare in today's multifaceted organizations. Providers at all levels are compelled to affiliate with others to function and thrive in such a complex environment, and the options for affiliation seem almost endless.

In this chapter, we will consider how we arrived at the current array of affiliation models. They did not emerge overnight; they are the result of literally decades of societal and economic issues and realities that have changed the healthcare landscape in America, including the increased involvement of state, local, and federal governments.

We learn from history; thus, we begin by looking back 50 years and working our way to the present. Some of the models we discuss in the following chapters have been around for years; they are merely repackaged to be more responsive to present-day settings. Others are newer and a reflection of the dynamics within our healthcare industry, which is still largely private-entity-based.

Additionally, our healthcare providers (mostly hospitals and health systems) are significantly represented as not-for-profit, tax-exempt entities. Physicians and related providers, if private, are likely for-profit entities, but they work closely across the aisle with not-for-profits. When they become fully affiliated/aligned with not-for-profit health systems, however, they may not be officially not-for-profit entities. Likewise, for-profit health systems should be considered within the various transactional structures of affiliation.

Finally, there is an abundance of private practicing physician groups and related ancillary service entities. Note: In this context, we define ancillary service entities as those that provide healthcare services directly to the provision of professional care, but ancillary services are in addition to (and billed as such) professional services. Examples include imaging, surgical, and diagnostic testing services.

With history as a basis, let's explore how the past has shaped our current (and projected future) landscape regarding affiliation models and associated transactions. By definition, we are broadening our consideration of transactional relationships to include physicians and hospitals/health systems; physicians with other physicians; physicians and health systems with for-profit investor entities, including private equity (PE) firms; and all other forms of potential affiliation, including insurance companies/payers. In short, the *universe* of potential partners in today's healthcare affiliation transactions has virtually no limitations.

FIGURE 1.1. Traditional Alignment Model Descriptions

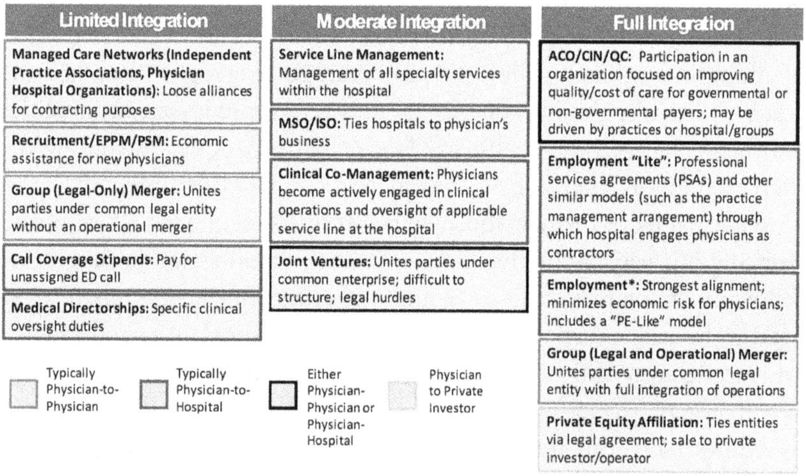

Limited Integration	Moderate Integration	Full Integration
Managed Care Networks (Independent Practice Associations, Physician Hospital Organizations): Loose alliances for contracting purposes	**Service Line Management:** Management of all specialty services within the hospital	**ACO/CIN/QC:** Participation in an organization focused on improving quality/cost of care for governmental or non-governmental payers; may be driven by practices or hospital/groups
Recruitment/EPPM/PSM: Economic assistance for new physicians	**MSO/ISO:** Ties hospitals to physician's business	**Employment "Lite":** Professional services agreements (PSAs) and other similar models (such as the practice management arrangement) through which hospital engages physicians as contractors
Group (Legal-Only) Merger: Unites parties under common legal entity without an operational merger	**Clinical Co-Management:** Physicians become actively engaged in clinical operations and oversight of applicable service line at the hospital	**Employment*:** Strongest alignment; minimizes economic risk for physicians; includes a "PE-Like" model
Call Coverage Stipends: Pay for unassigned ED call	**Joint Ventures:** Unites parties under common enterprise; difficult to structure; legal hurdles	**Group (Legal and Operational) Merger:** Unites parties under common legal entity with full integration of operations
Medical Directorships: Specific clinical oversight duties		**Private Equity Affiliation:** Ties entities via legal agreement; sale to private investor/operator

Legend: Typically Physician-to-Physician; Typically Physician-to-Hospital; Either Physician-Physician or Physician-Hospital; Physician to Private Investor

* *Includes the Physician Enterprise Model (PEM) and the Group Practice Subsidiary (GPS) model both of which allow the practice entity to remain intact even after employment of the physicians by the hospital*

Figure 1.1 serves as the foundation for this discussion and is referenced in detail as we explore the specific models presented throughout this book. Moreover, all these examples are applicable as we consider the history of transactional affiliation models. Many are not new or untried, though some are more recently developed and incorporated in the transactional affiliation structures.

Now, let's take a walk down memory lane and consider how our healthcare system has changed in the context of physicians and related providers and their affiliation structures over the past 50 years.

THE 1970s AND 1980s

We group these two decades because they have similar characteristics relative to affiliation transaction models and structures. The U.S. economy during the 1970s was somewhat volatile, with high interest rates and inflationary economic trends. The economy slowed in the latter part of the 1970s, with inflation and interest rates often reaching double digits. Economic trends improved in the 1980s, allowing greater affluence and better financial times. Overall, the healthcare industry mirrored these trends.

With this economic backdrop, the relationships between healthcare providers—physicians and hospitals/health systems—were mostly at arm's length. Transactional integration was rare. Most physicians were in private practice; many were in small groups or solo practices. Physicians who were just out of training and ready to start their career in medicine generally considered two options: working within a private group with aspirations to become a partner within that group or starting a solo practice.

Although some physicians practiced in larger groups, little emphasis was placed on mergers. The reimbursement model was fee-for-service, though some areas of the country introduced risk-based contracts tied mostly to capitated models, also called managed care, in the late 1980s. Typically, the capitation models were with primary care; specialists were rarely involved in capitation arrangements. (See "A Short History of Managed Care" in the sidebar.)

A SHORT HISTORY OF MANAGED CARE

Government intervention to control cost in the healthcare market has a long history. The Health Maintenance Organization Act of 1973 directly promoted the development of HMOs. In the 1980s, the prospective payment system (PPS) for Medicare was introduced in an effort to curtail healthcare costs in hospitals. Hospitals were reimbursed a pre-determined amount for each diagnostic-related group (DRG). DRGs were intended to motivate hospitals to increase efficiency and minimize unnecessary spending, as they would only be reimbursed a set amount for each diagnostic category. To provide a way of measuring provider efficiency by DRG category, resource-based relative value units (RBRVU) were introduced. Each RBRVU corresponded to a DRG. RBRVUs, however, continued to reimburse physician providers on a fee-for-service basis and reflected a highly complex set of calculations.

In the 1990s, private organizations and employers sponsored HMOs, PPOs, and physician hospital organizations (PHOs) as part of their managed-care efforts to reduce costs by eliminating provider incentives for inappropriate care and excess productivity. Many MCOs entered capitated arrangements with contracted physicians, wherein such providers would receive a fixed amount per patient month per member (PMPM). Capitation was intended to emphasize primary care as central to improving healthcare and keeping hospital costs under the budgeted amount.

Yet capitation created a perverse financial motive to deny access to care and limit utilization, which was detrimental to patients. Because payment was not tied to outcomes, capitation arguably encouraged providers to cut spending without enough concern for patient welfare.

"A Short History of Managed Care." Medical Device and Diagnostic Industry, September 15, 2011. https://www.mddionline.com/short-history-managed-care. Accessed January 26, 2020.

Hospitals were keenly aware of the need to work with physicians and allied healthcare providers, but the relationship was mostly through medical staff membership and more distant affiliations. Referring to Figure 1.1, the relationships among physicians and hospitals are captured in the Limited Integration column. Many physicians were members of medical staffs of various hospitals—usually competing facilities. Physicians may have looked to hospitals for financial assistance but usually in the context of recruitment support and/or medical directorships and possibly some compensation for specific contracted services, depending on the specialty and overall needs of the hospital. There were few mega-groups. Some multi-specialty groups existed and even a few larger single-specialty groups; however, private practicing physicians' ability to realize a level of reimbursement that allowed them an acceptable bottom line (i.e., take-home pay) left few desiring anything more than an at-arm's-length relationship with hospitals. Similarly, hospitals saw no pressing need to employ or closely integrate with physicians.

HOSPITAL OF YESTERDAY: THE BIGGEST CHANGES IN HEALTHCARE

In years past, the hospital experience included lengthy stays, severe blind spots in prevention, and a lack of patient respect, according to medical historians and health care professionals.

https://health.usnews.com/health-news/hospital-of-tomorrow/articles/2014/07/15/hospital-of-yesterday-the-biggest-changes-in-health-care

Hospitals were more concerned about medical staff relations and overall responsiveness to their physicians who often had a choice of which competitive hospital facility to work with and refer their patients to. Consequently, hospitals became acutely aware of the need to provide *customer service* to private physician groups through improved responsiveness and support of the patients the physicians admitted to the hospital, which was not the typical model at the time (see "Hospital of Yesterday: The Biggest Changes in Healthcare" sidebar). Fewer outpatient services were provided than is currently the case. The delivery of inpatient services that called for inpatient stays was still the dominant form of care, especially in surgical cases (see "Long Stays" sidebar.)

LONG STAYS

It once was common for a woman to spend 10 days in the hospital after giving birth, rather than today's more-standard 24-hour turnaround. Other health care services also came with long hospital stays: Dr. Peter Kernahan, a retired physician and medical historian, says when he started his residency in the late 1970s, a patient with a hernia could spend four days in the hospital after an operation. Now, the surgery is performed on an outpatient basis.

https://health.usnews.com/health-news/hospital-of-tomorrow/articles/2014/07/15/hospital-of-yesterday-the-biggest-changes-in-health-care

Moreover, physicians were able to realize acceptable incomes without providing diagnostic imaging and surgical services outside of the hospital (i.e., within their practice imaging center, surgery center, etc., as a direct competitor). This created an unwritten—and at that time, reasonable—line of demarcation between the services hospitals performed and those of physician groups. Physician groups concentrated on providing professional services and billing and collecting for them, which was enough to meet their financial obligations and compensation requirements. Hospitals understood their boundaries and placed more emphasis on inpatient revenue while providing virtually all the ancillary services, such as imaging, surgical, other diagnostic testing, durable medical equipment, pharmacy, etc. The boundaries were fairly clear-cut.

As for reimbursement from third-party payers, while some risk-based contracts started to develop in the latter part of the 1980s, creating more interest in physician-hospital affiliation in the 1990s, reimbursement was primarily fee-for-service or fee-for-*volume,* and rates were acceptable because the cost of care was manageable. The most significant expenses in private medical practices were personnel compensation and benefits, as is the case today. During the 1970s and 1980s, however, personnel expenses were manageable and did not place undue stress on the bottom line.

A look back at the 1970s and 1980s might cause us to wish to return to a time when healthcare was much easier to navigate, both economically and operationally. Traditional boundaries were set for physicians and hospitals with little interest in investors for either. Despite the economic challenges and aggressive inflationary trends during the late 1970s, hospitals and physicians were able to coexist as entirely separate entities. Still, the two had to work together, but not by forming legal affiliation models such as those noted in Figure 1.1 under the Moderate and Full Integration categories.

THE 1990s

The 1990s was a decade that experienced the most significant paradigm shift in physician practice structures that had ever occurred in U.S. history. Shortly after his election in 1992, President Clinton appointed a healthcare reform task force to develop a proposal for providing healthcare benefits for all American citizens and legal residents. The concept introduced the increasing possibility of a government takeover of the U.S. healthcare system.

Though this takeover did not materialize, it did create a significant shift in attitudes among both physicians and health systems. That shift led physicians to look to hospitals for employment and led hospitals to consider forming what was at that time termed *integrated delivery systems*. These integrated delivery systems were intended to be a response to not only the government attempts for greater participation in healthcare delivery system, but other private insurers' attempts to change the reimbursement structure. As such, the importance of physicians, particularly primary care physicians, leading the entry point to healthcare for many patients and initiating the adoption of a *gatekeeper* concept emerged.

Reimbursement changed to carry out these concepts wherein employers, while still maintaining responsibility for their employees' healthcare insurance, agreed to manage the delivery of healthcare via the primary care provider gatekeeper concepts and the reimbursement structure on a per-member-per-month capitated basis.

This rush to change the reimbursement structure, along with the anticipated possible change in the government's role in healthcare in the United States, led to a perfect storm in which many hospitals/health systems attempted to form networks of integrated providers. They acquired multiple practices and recruited many physicians directly out of training into employment to build their networks.

An interesting series of events unfolded pertaining to physician-hospital affiliation. Based on the rules and regulations surrounding physicians' referrals to hospitals, scrutiny heightened concerning the "purchasing" of those referrals or inurement to those physicians in return for their referrals. While the rules and regulations had been in place for some time, the attention escalated. Many transactions during the early 1990s involved hospitals purchasing physician practices for significantly high amounts of upfront money couched as goodwill. Further, the post-transaction compensation employment structure was lucrative. Subsequently, many misguided transactions were made that were destined to fail.

Many acquisitions by health systems did not render favorable results regarding the working relationship and the economic ramifications of the entire transaction. Hospitals paid too much for too little work and too few incentives for the physicians to be productive after the deal settled. Perhaps the crowning blow of this challenging situation was that the Clinton administration failed in its attempt to convey more power to the government in the administration of healthcare.

Also, capitation and risk-based contracting were collectively unpopular. Providers, payers, and hospitals (the most crucial component) failed miserably in managing the practices that they purchased. Although managing and operating a medical practice is significantly different from managing and administering a hospital, many hospitals tried to run practices in the same way they managed their hospital, which typically, they did well.

By the end of the 1990s, many health systems' administrations and boards had concluded that the employment model of alignment/affiliation with physicians was unnecessary for strategic and tactical reasons, and it was impractical for economic and return-on-investment purposes. Therefore, by the close of the decade and early into the 21st century, many health systems stepped away from the physician employment/integrated model. Though they separated, they still attempted to maintain relationships and, in many cases, provided physicians "a soft landing" back into private practice.

Another dynamic that developed in this decade was the concept of *physician practice management companies* (PPMCs). The business basis of PPMCs was to emphasize the role of the primary care provider. As such, these providers would sell their practices—again, for somewhat inflated values in exchange for management contracts. Also, a portion of the sale of the practice was attributable to and applied to either stock rights or direct equity in the management company. The hope was that the PPMC would be successful and ultimately, the value of the equity attributable to the practice would be exchanged in a public offering for a premium price. This arrangement would also address some of the issues relative to aggregation and risk-based contracting as the PPMCs were better equipped to manage risks within their infrastructures; at least, that was the theory.

Generally, the PPMCs did a good job managing the practices. However, because the industry did not shift and there was not enough profit left for the physicians and for the PPMC, or to attract the public investors to buy-in, most PPMCs were defunct by the end of the decade. Indeed, the PPMC industry probably had the shortest life span in the history of U.S. healthcare.

Although the close of the 1990s left many unanswered questions, many physicians were back in private practice, looking to aggregate through mergers into larger groups. The government was unsettled as to how to deal with healthcare reform; the payers were unsure about reimbursement, though they continued to focus on fee-for-service with little risk-based contracting; and the entire provider base faced many unknowns after several affiliation models (i.e., employment, PPMC aggregation, group mergers, etc.) had in essence failed.

THE 21ST CENTURY—FIRST DECADE

Physician affiliation transactions continued to evolve into the new century. On the heels of the late 1990s when many deals were undone, especially between hospitals and physicians, the number of new transactions and/or extensions of existing ones were minimal. Further, the disengagement of many original transactions between physicians and hospitals continued.

The tragic attacks on September 11, 2001, negatively affected the U.S. economy and every industry in America. Physician groups continued to look at their options for the future with special note toward some hospital-alignment transactions and some groups increasing in size through mergers. Fee-for-service was still the preferred reimbursement structure and reimbursement itself was reasonably good. The government continued to evaluate reimbursement relative to Medicare and gave only small increases on a year-to-year basis.

Some specific events near the end of the decade drove certain specialties to greater alignment, most notably cardiology. The government reduced reimbursement to private cardiology practices for in-practice imaging and diagnostic testing. Reimbursements for nuclear studies, echocardiograms, etc., were reduced significantly, though these cuts did not apply for such services performed within hospitals and/or outpatient hospital departments.

With these changes, many cardiologists in private practice shifted their focus toward alignment transactions with hospitals. This change was driven by their dependency on revenue from ancillary services such as nuclear studies and echoes administered in their private practice. Those who had developed a significant percentage of their overall revenue in these areas were often the first to seek an affiliation with a hospital. This illustrates how a specific paradigm shift in reimbursement can have a major effect on affiliation transactions, especially among hospitals and physician groups.

Another innovative concept that surfaced toward the end of the first decade of the 21st century was the introduction of professional services agreements (PSAs) as a form of affiliation/alignment in place of employment. These PSAs took on various forms and mainly consisted of IRS-1099 relationships among physician groups and hospitals. Cardiology transactions were often consummated via a PSA structure, though most were still under a traditional employment model. (We will consider the origins of PSA transactions and their relationship to alignment structures in Chapter 6).

The Obama administration, which came into office in 2009, campaigned that healthcare reform would be a major part of its first administration. With the Democrats in control of both the House and the Senate, Obamacare (officially, The Patient Protection and Affordable Care Act [PPACA] and referred to as the Affordable Care Act [ACA]; see "Obamacare" sidebar) was passed and signed into law on March 23, 2010. Interestingly, this created a new opportunity for physicians, hospitals, and others for various forms of affiliation. The law called for few changes during its first years, but with more changes prescribed toward the end of President Obama's second administration (2014 and beyond). The ACA was to emphasize forms of reimbursement related to *value-based* as opposed to *volume-based* payments, which are still on the horizon. While value-based reimbursement (VBR) includes various areas of non-fee-for-volume payments tied to cost savings, quality, and overall efficiency of care, in truth, the success of the ACA is limited, if it exists at all. Moreover, the affiliation models tied to volume-based reimbursement have yet to take shape to any degree.

OBAMACARE

The Patient Protection and **Affordable Care Act** (PPACA), often shortened to the **Affordable Care Act** (ACA) or nicknamed Obamacare, is a United States federal statute enacted by the 111th United States Congress and signed into law by President Barack Obama on March 23, 2010.

Some additional new models have formed, including clinical co-management agreements (CCMAs). CCMAs emphasize the aggregation of resources within specific specialties wherein hospitals and physicians can gather to manage the throughput of services, especially for a particular specialty. Such specialties as heart care, cancer care, musculoskeletal care, etc., have experienced success within CCMA structures (see Chapter 10 for more discussion).

At the close of the first decade of the 21st century, the ACA ranked as the highest concern and most uncertain aspect of our healthcare system regarding how to best deal with the future and, specifically, alignment/affiliation transactions. During this period, relatively few transactions were completed, except in cardiology or other areas more subject to fee-for-service changes, not value-based changes. Most providers took a wait-and-see attitude about how future events would unfold. Most parties agreed, however, that VBR, population health management (PHM), and related initiatives would be forthcoming. The second decade of the 21st century proved otherwise.

THE 21ST CENTURY—SECOND DECADE

Nearing completion of a second decade of the new century, the number and variety of affiliation structures continue to evolve, generating a full range of transactions. In Figure 1.1, we noted some innovative structures under consideration from which transactions have resulted.

One of the areas of growth is physician practices affiliating with *private equity* (PE)-backed or directly owned entities. These models assume a variety of structures, including management services and outright equity participation/ownership. We discuss this dynamic form of affiliation in Chapter 8.

A somewhat newer unproven model, the *private equity-like structure*, is explored in Chapter 9. While it requires more evaluation and testing, it may have limited appeal among health systems and larger private groups that would typically be interested in a PE transaction. The PE-like model tries to offset the PE transaction itself as a viable alternative for alignment among larger single- and multi-specialty groups and health systems. (See Chapter 9 for further discussion.)

In the second decade of this century, we are seeing renewals of existing agreements. These *second-generation* transactions and affiliations have become interesting in the context of the changes that have resulted. For example, the first-generation deals may have considered a traditional work relative value unit (wRVU) incentive model for compensation, which could apply for both PSA and employment models. The second-generation renewal models place more emphasis on value-based/quality-based metrics and incentives and less emphasis on production in wRVUs and related metrics. Second-generation models reflect both market realities and the supply/demand situations.

Further, the financial experiences of the employer/contractor during the first-generation model are a factor in play. Many of the first-generation deals resulted in higher losses to the employer than anticipated. Thus, the second generations are tightening the terms, conditions, and compensation parameters over the initial agreements. (See Chapter 2 for further discussion.)

Another characteristic of the current decade is an increase in PSA transactions. Initially, PSAs were frowned upon, especially by hospitals who did not see the value compared to employment, mainly due to the relative independence and autonomy that the practice retained. As more PSAs were implemented, this issue became less significant when the practices responded well to this structure. We believe that PSAs will continue to be a prominent form of affiliation, although it is full alignment, as noted in Figure 1.1. (See Chapter 6 for further discussion.)

Mergers are another consideration for groups that want to remain private. These are discussed in greater detail in Chapter 13 and to some extent, Chapter 14. Group mergers will continue to be popular, but we add a word of caution: Pulling together disparate groups (and to some degree, cultures) is a challenging undertaking. In Chapter 13, we discuss the various forms of mergers. We also address the significant effect the level of operational merging has on whether a merger can occur.

Clinically integrated networks (CINs) have begun to gain popularity. CINs are a derivative of value-based reimbursement/PHM and are in response to the ACA and related changes in reimbursement structures (i.e., moving from strictly fee-for-volume to fee-for-value). CINs often are a derivative of original physician-hospital organizations (PHOs) and/or independent physician associations (IPAs) that have moved into and are scrutinized to be legally structured as clinically integrated organizations (CIOs). This allows for collective marketing and other joint efforts, including payer contracting (perhaps the greatest value of all) of the CIN. Chapter 12 delves into CINs and VBR affiliation models in much more detail.

Joint equity ventures are common. They include hospitals, private investors, and/or physician groups and often can include all three major entities. They can encompass everything from medical office buildings and other real estate to ancillary services and, to some extent, practice clinics, surgery centers, and imaging centers. Joint equity ventures are important to explore, especially when employment or other forms of full alignment are not of interest or viable. Chapter 7 reviews joint equity ventures in detail.

Thus, the second decade of the 21st century offers a wide variety of affiliation models in response to the market and the healthcare industry today. There is a somewhat wait-and-see attitude toward VBR and related population health models, but there also is a continued emphasis (if not an absolute requirement) on cost controls and overall improved efficiencies plus throughput of clinical care.

These models all point to *cost controls*, *high quality*, and *operational efficiency*. We believe that the healthcare industry has heard the message that the consumer as well as the government (and private paying insurance companies) expect high levels of quality and demand improved performance in controlling costs and delivering services efficiently. Whatever the form of affiliation, now and in the future, these three factors are essential.

Finally, we emphasize that the level of government involvement and scrutiny in healthcare regulatory requirements is at its highest level in history. No matter the structure, whether a health system, for-profit or not-for-profit, private equity entity, private physician group, etc., all must adhere and continually comply with government requirements. Many requirements revolve around the transaction of affiliation addressed in this book. Those transactions among health systems and physicians and other providers are subject to the highest scrutiny, and no one is immune from government regulatory compliance. This pertains to everything from anti-trust legislation to physician compensation, private inurement relative to physician referrals, valuation considerations, compensation, and fair market value/commercially reasonable parameters. Adherence to all regulatory matters is the requirement for not-for-profit, tax-exempt status to be in full compliance.

SUMMARY

History is an important teacher for those making plans. Understanding the rich history of healthcare over the past five decades relative to physicians, hospitals, and other entity affiliation models will help everyone make sound decisions in the future. In this chapter, we have laid the foundation for the remainder of the book. Let us now move on and drill down on these individual models and consider other relevant discussion points.

CHAPTER 2

Evolution of Economics of Physician Affiliation Models

Using Chapter 1 as a springboard, a continuation of a brief history of reform efforts and their effect on the marketplace competition can help us understand how the economics of physician affiliation models have evolved. This discussion includes the state of the healthcare industry through the 1980s, the managed competition theory dominating much of the 1990s' healthcare reform debate, consolidation and reforms in the insurance industry in the 2000s, and current healthcare reform efforts and consolidation of providers. We then will explore how these changing environments have impacted specific alignment models and the underlying economics of them.

PRE-1990s

Several guiding principles dominated the U.S. healthcare system up through the 1980s. As summarized by Stanford University professor Alain Enthoven, these included:

1. Free choice of doctor by the patient;
2. Free choice of treatment by the doctor;
3. Direct negotiation between doctor and patient regarding fees;
4. Fee-for-service payment; and
5. Solo or small, single-specialty group practice.[1]

Many in the industry described these principles as anti-competitive, arguing that limited patient knowledge, limited payer bargaining power, and mutual coercion through control of referrals ultimately hurt consumers. These arguments were the primary drivers behind healthcare reform efforts in the 1990s.

MANAGED CARE AND MANAGED COMPETITION

Though its roots date back to the early 1900s, managed care was spurred by the enactment of the Health Maintenance Organization Act of 1973. Managed care was intended to reduce healthcare costs by emphasizing treatment planning and quality management, focusing on having the most appropriate care provided in the most appropriate setting, and managing patients through the continuum of care. Initiatives implemented through managed care include:

- Incentives for physicians and patients to select less costly forms of care;
- Programs for reviewing the medical necessity of specific services;
- Increased beneficiary cost-sharing;
- Controls on inpatient admissions and lengths of stay;
- Cost-sharing incentives for outpatient surgery;
- Selective contracting with healthcare providers; and
- The intensive management of high-cost healthcare cases.

A major push to reform the healthcare industry began in the 1990s. Managed competition was the dominant model for change and the primary basis upon which the Clinton administration's healthcare reform proposal, the American Health Security Act of 1993, was built. At its core, managed competition is a theory of healthcare delivery services that holds that the quality and efficiency of such services would improve if, in a market controlled by the federal government, independent groups had to compete for healthcare consumers.

As envisioned, competing healthcare entities, particularly payers, were to be monitored by a supervisory structure that established equitable rules, created price-elastic demand, and avoided uncompensated risk selection. The model represented a combination of competitive and regulatory strategies to achieve maximum value for consumers and providers compatible with many Americans' preference for pluralism, individual choice and responsibility, and universal coverage.

When Clinton's healthcare reform efforts collapsed in 1994, many employers quickly turned to health maintenance organization (HMO) plans. From 1993 to 1996, the HMO market share rose from 21% to 31% (see Figure 2.1).

Although Clinton's American Health Security Act of 1993 was declared dead in the Senate in late 1994, other major healthcare legisla-

FIGURE 2.1. Market Shares, 1988–2001

Market Shares	1988	1993	1996	1998	2001
Conventional	73%	46%	27%	14%	7%
Health Maintenance Organization (HMO)	16%	21%	31%	27%	24%
Preferred Provider Organization (PPO)	11%	26%	28%	35%	46%
Point-of-Service (POS)	0%	7%	14%	24%	23%

Source: The Kaiser Family Foundation and the Health Research and Educational Trust (2004).

tion was passed. Among the notable reforms was the Health Insurance Portability and Accountability Act (HIPAA), a significant expansion of the Stark physician self-referral law (Stark II), and the State Children's Health Insurance Program (S-CHIP).

Initially, managed-care programs seemed to slow the pace of year-over-year healthcare expenditure increases. Still, healthcare expenditures grew an average of 1.67% faster than GDP between 1994 and 1999. However, in 2000 and 2001, the pace of healthcare spending increases ticked up drastically, rising 3.0% and 7.5% (see Figure 2.2). Hospitals and health systems started realizing significant losses on their practice acquisitions, and many of the managed-care integration efforts of the era collapsed.

FIGURE 2.2. Healthcare Expenditures, 1994–2001

Year	GDP	Healthcare Expenditures	Difference
1994	4.00%	5.50%	1.50%
1995	2.70%	5.60%	2.90%
1996	3.80%	5.20%	1.40%
1997	4.40%	5.70%	1.30%
1998	4.50%	5.80%	1.30%
1999	4.80%	6.40%	1.60%
2000	4.10%	7.10%	3.00%
2001	1.00%	8.50%	7.50%

Source: The Bureau of Economic Analysis, U.S. Department of Commerce

INDUSTRY CONSOLIDATION AND DIVESTITURE

As previously noted, many physicians historically practiced independently or as part of small, single-specialty groups competing with one another, allied perhaps only with the hospital(s) to which they referred patients. As Hoangmai Pham and Paul Ginsberg described, primary care physicians (PCPs) and many specialists relied on the office as their base of operations, where they provided consultations, ongoing ambulatory care, minor tests, and electrocardiograms. Hospitals were physicians' workshops, a place where they provided major procedures and services that were more technology-dependent or where PCPs and cognitive specialists managed care for patients requiring hospital admission. Traditionally, because the hospital housed the workshop, it received remuneration from payers to cover staff and facility expenses, while physicians received fees for the professional services they provided there.[2]

Through the 1980s and 1990s, declining Medicare reimbursement introduced with the prospective payment system, the arrival of managed care and healthcare reform efforts, and decreasing demand for hospital beds as medical services increasingly shifted to the outpatient setting all combined to ignite a flurry of consolidation in the healthcare industry, including physician practice acquisitions by hospitals, health systems, and large integrated groups. However, with sharp rises in healthcare costs and the collapse of many managed care-driven efforts, integrated systems began experiencing significant financial losses on physician acquisitions, leading to a wave of physician practice divestitures in the 2000s.

During the past few years, several legislative initiatives have reignited consolidation efforts. The advent of accountable care organizations (ACOs) and patient-centered medical homes, increasing costs of maintaining physician practices, rising regulatory scrutiny, and new technology demands such as electronic medical records and ICD-10 conversion are all driving this latest round of consolidation. Also contributing are the changing physician demographics and priorities (i.e., increasing numbers of older physicians and preferences of younger physicians both leading to a greater emphasis on work-life balance).

This wave of consolidation has shaped the healthcare industry in new ways. Many regulations designed to reign in the competition have been altered, such as Stark/Anti-Kickback and anti-trust waivers for ACOs.

The increasing push for greater coordination of care among providers is also driving new alignment between hospitals and physicians.

THE DESIRE TO ALIGN

From the physician's perspective, alignment in an era of change is an attractive way to obtain greater security and stability. While many look to employment as an option, larger physician groups especially are not rushing in that direction. These groups often find that contractual relationships, such as professional service agreements and CCMAs, may be more beneficial than employment.

From the hospital perspective, finding methods to align beyond employment may be attractive due to economic feasibility and the ability to share financial risk equally with the physician group. Hospitals and health systems also commonly are developing a pluralistic approach to alignment, exploring, and implementing many different alignment models simultaneously.

EVOLUTION OF ECONOMICS AND STRUCTURES

Compared with the consolidation wave of the 1990s, economic terms and transaction structures continue to be refined. In the current swell of consolidation and alignment, more weight is being placed on realistic transaction values and remuneration for services—those that are within fair market value and commercial reasonableness parameters. Hospitals also are increasingly introducing non-productivity measures and incentives tied to both cost controls and quality outcomes. Further, hospitals are recognizing the value of physicians as leaders and are moving governance initiatives to a dyad structure where physicians are empowered in the decision-making process within hospitals, allowing them to function more as partners than as adversaries, as they sometimes operated historically.

During the past 20 years, hospital-physician agreements under all alignment models have become more uniform and less negotiable from one physician to the next. At a more granular level, trends towards shorter contracts are also being observed. While three-year terms were once standard (and are still quite common), many healthcare organizations and practices are moving toward one-year, renewable contracts—slowly shifting closer to the at-will structures of non-physician staff and employees.

SUMMARY

In this chapter, we have used the universal concepts of the evolution of healthcare, as denoted in Chapter One, and developed more detail about the economic drivers that affect current-day alignment options between physicians and health systems. One subtle observation is the increase in uniformity in the arrangements and models—the need for standardization. Another is the conviction that the systems must work collaboratively to survive and thrive in the marketplace. Decisions must make sense economically.

The following chapters will explore the reasons for affiliation and individual models in more detail.

REFERENCES

1. Enthoven AC. The History and Principles of Managed Competition. *Health Affairs.* 1993;12 Suppl. 24-48. https://doi.org/10.1377/hlthaff.12.suppl_1.24
2. Pham HH and Ginsberg PB. Unhealthy Trends: The Future of Physician Services. *Health Affairs.* 2007; 26(6):1587, 1589.

CHAPTER 3

Reasons for Affiliation

The increase in physician affiliations is not without explanation. The reasons for creating affiliations are substantiated repeatedly and continue to be supported. This chapter details these considerations, especially relative to current strategies, and paves the way for the remainder of the discussions.

DRIVERS FOR AFFILIATION

The drivers for affiliation are as varied as the models for affiliation themselves. Seemingly, every transaction that closes, whether among physicians or between physicians and hospitals, has a different reason for inception. Some affiliations are necessary to ensure continued operational success, some are hedges against future changes, and yet others are based on financial motives. The overarching reason for most affiliations, however, is related to one of four primary drivers: strategic, operational, financial, or environmental, as denoted in Figure 3.1.

FIGURE 3.1. Primary Drivers for Affiliation

Strategic	Operational
Financial	Environmental

Each driver is considered in greater detail in this chapter.

Strategic Drivers

Strategic drivers can encompass patient care, growth, competition, physician engagement, value-based reimbursement, and expansion of the market base.

Better Care of Patients. Within the healthcare industry, patients often are seen as the "True North." (Note: True North is a key concept in Lean process improvement. It might be viewed as a mission statement, a reflection of the purpose of the organization, and the foundation of a strategic plan.) Patients and their needs and interests should be top of mind and at the forefront of decision making.

For many organizations, providing improved care to patients and better meeting their needs are sufficient reasons for pursuing an affiliation. An example is the solo physician practice. Here, (1) patients have limited access with only one provider to see all the patients, (2) with few or no ancillaries that allow patients convenient access to comprehensive testing, and (3) using outdated technology due to the inherent cost of obtaining new equipment.

This physician joins a health system that can bring the solo provider and, equally as important, all the provider's patients, into a network that has the support structures the solo practice lacked. For practices of this type, taking better care of patients requires aligning with another entity that has greater capacity and resources to care for patients more completely.

Growth. The opportunity for growth is supported by most successful affiliations. In effective affiliations, the desired algebra is no longer 1 + 1 = 2, but rather, 1 + 1 = 3. But how is this possible? Affiliations combine resources that collectively support expansion, whether that is the ability to support additional providers, the skilled resources to develop new service lines, or the capital for real estate expansion. The multiplier effect that affiliation affords makes multiple forms of growth possible.

Competitive Advantage. Economist and author Michael Porter identified three ways organizations can maintain a competitive advantage:

1. Cost leadership – providing valued services at a lower cost;
2. Differentiation – providing better services than the competition; and
3. Focus – best meeting the target audience's needs.[1]

Interestingly, within healthcare, affiliations can support all three of Porter's ways of creating and maintaining a competitive advantage. For example, a health system that develops a large employed provider group through affiliations, and then uses it as a vehicle to provide its employees high-quality, low-cost care at a discounted rate, is an excellent example of cost leadership.

Concerning differentiation, recruiting a highly trained and heavily practiced neurosurgeon could be a massive differentiator for some hospitals. Regarding focus, bringing together orthopedic surgeons, physical therapists, and skilled nursing providers in a single affiliated model in a community with an average population age of 71 could also be one effective method for maintaining a competitive advantage. However, all those scenarios first require affiliation.

Physician Engagement. Physician engagement (and its antonym, physician burnout) is one of the most frequently discussed topics in healthcare literature today. The research, including that of the Mayo Clinic, indicates that creating a sense of community at work increases physician engagement. More specifically, peer support helps physicians navigate challenges and reduces their risk of burnout.[2] This peer support is another form of affiliation, and although it may be less formal than structures such as employment, it remains an important form of affiliation, particularly in this era of increasing physician burnout. Keeping physicians connected to their peers as a way to increase engagement is another reason for affiliation.

Adapting to the Value-Based Reimbursement (VBR) Environment. The belief that strength comes in numbers has spread steadily since the advent of the VBR era. Structures such as ACOs and CINs, which bring together disparate entities to function as a single operating unit, both exemplify the "strength-in-numbers" concept and underscore the notion that being successful in VBR requires affiliated unified entities.

Access to Larger Customer Base. While access to more providers, more capital, and more space are all reasons for affiliation, access to more customers is another driver. Although in healthcare, customers typically are referred to as patients, the fact is that healthcare entities sometimes need more customers/patients to make their business hum, and affiliations can provide access to a larger customer base. For example, the vertical integration in organizations such as Kaiser Permanente and Intermountain Health creates opportunities across the hospital, medical group, and payer enterprises.

Operational Drivers

Operational efficiency, leadership, integrated electronic medical records (EMRs), physician involvement, and ancillary services are the primary operational drivers of affiliation.

Operational Efficiency. If you have ever peeked inside a restaurant kitchen, you may have noticed the organization of the foods and spices. Typically, fresh produce, meats, and dairy products are stored in separate areas. Putting like things together in the proper place creates efficiency, and as most successful restaurants know, efficiency is key in getting fresh, hot food to hungry diners. This efficiency is also what many affiliations seek.

An example in healthcare is the co-location of specialties. A common goal is that after affiliation (and particularly once the transaction has yielded a critical mass of providers), all specialty providers will be relocated, particularly if they previously were in individual siloes across myriad facilities. Co-locating providers/specialties/services in a logical order generates the operational efficiencies that yield the best possible results. This strategy was not viable until affiliation aligned the interests of the parties and made it worth their while (strategically, operationally, and/or financially) to relocate.

Dedicated Administrative Leadership. Many organizations, particularly private practices, use affiliation to access a deeper bench of administrative resources. Typically, with affiliation comes the opportunity to use or bolster the administrative team, either through dyad leadership or by creating an enhanced support team with differing levels of responsibility.

For example, rather than having a single office manager who oversees all operations, affiliation with a larger entity could afford access to an administrative CEO as well as director- and manager-level resources who are focused on specific strategic areas throughout the organization. Until they become affiliated with a larger entity, it can be difficult for smaller practices to recruit or afford that level of administrative leadership.

Integrated Electronic Medical Record (EMR). Imagine reading a book in which every other page has been ripped out. While you may be able to understand the overall plot, you would most assuredly lose essential details that add flavor, richness, and context for the story. Now, imagine you are a physician who does not have access to every page of a patient's story because you do not have access to their entire medical history.

Without interoperable EMRs, physicians often feel as though they are reading a patient's story but without key pages. This missing information is another reason for affiliation. Accessing complete patient records seamlessly, as is achieved with interoperable EMRs available post-affiliation, enhances patient care, and improves safety and quality.

Opportunities for Physician Leadership. A growing number of physicians have an interest in fulfilling leadership duties outside the delivery of clinical care (such as chief medical officer, chief quality officer, or physician executive). Between running a business and seeing patients, this role is not always feasible. Nevertheless, affiliation can afford physicians an opportunity to transition some oversight of their business to their strategic partner, thus freeing them up to take leadership positions that would not otherwise be possible.

Expansion of Locations, Services, Ancillaries. One of the most fundamental reasons for affiliation is the opportunity to expand. As discussed throughout this chapter, affiliation makes expansion possible in myriad ways, including expansion into new locations (i.e., geographic markets), facilities, and service offerings.

Financial Drivers

The financial drivers that affect affiliation are the increase in returns, cost controls, access to capital, and economies of scale.

Financial Return. While some organizations pursue affiliation for purely strategic reasons, it is much more common that the arrangement also is accompanied by an expectation for improved financial performance. Since alliances can be costly, most organizations do not enter into them by chance. Instead, they plan carefully to determine what return is available for that initial investment; in many cases, if there is no potential return, the planning activities end and the transaction ceases.

With many organizations operating with margins in the range of 1–4%, the cost of the affiliation must yield some return. However, improved returns are decidedly possible, with many organizations realizing up to a 200x return on their investment, particularly when coupled by additional providers who support the initiative.

Cost Control. Since healthcare is a "people" business, emphasizing cost control as a reason for affiliation can be an emotionally charged issue. Reductions in force and eliminating positions are difficult choices, yet salaries are the most significant expense for nearly every healthcare entity and as such, must be considered seriously. When presented as part of an affiliation transaction, cost-control measures are still tricky, but they provide an opportunity for rightsizing that may otherwise have been too politically charged to accomplish.

Access to Capital. One of the reasons private equity (PE) backing has become increasingly popular in the healthcare industry is the infusion of capital that can accompany it. For some organizations limited by available dollars, the removal of that constraint allows them to flourish. Thus, having greater access to capital through the backing of PE or by having access to higher debt financing with increased available collateral (as often occurs in affiliation) is another key reason organizations look to affiliate.

Economies of Scale. There is a disconnect in the economies of scale believed possible and those actually achieved as a result of affiliation. One of the most significant economies of scale that results from healthcare affiliations is group purchasing—leveraging the collective size of two or more affiliated organizations in their purchasing power. Although this benefit may seem insignificant, achieving economies of scale is difficult and many healthcare affiliations fail to achieve them.

Environmental Drivers

Competition in the marketplace, marketing strength, payer pressures, succession planning, recruitment, and attrition are significant environmental drivers of affiliation.

Response to Market Competition. Long gone are the days when leadership at competing hospitals in a market would strike a gentleman's agreement on which key services they would each pursue. In today's world, it seems that every hospital wants to be recognized as the heart hospital, the cancer center, the woman/baby pavilion, as do their competitors across town. This rivalry pressures organizations to build or buy partnerships to remain relevant in their market.

Many hospitals affiliate because their competitors affiliate and they do not want to be without a partner. Thus, affiliation is a robust method for responding to market competition as it supports both the "build" and "buy" strategies.

Building Market Strength. While opposing market competition drives affiliation, so too does building market strength. This strength refers to the alignment of interests and subsequent aggregation of entities within a particular market, usually as a play for dominance across a region or state or as a defensive measure against encroaching competition.

The consolidation of Greenville Health System and Palmetto Health is an example. The two systems joined to become the largest not-for-profit health organization in South Carolina (https://www.prismahealth.org), which some suspect was a way to keep Atrium Health from taking over the state. In this case, rather than competing separately, the organizations decided to come together to face a mutual foe.

Meeting Payer Pressures. The narrowing of networks is a real fear for many organizations. Similar to what health systems have done, as payers create narrow networks, some providers/organizations will participate while others will not. The result is many more provider-payer affiliations. Look no further than one of UnitedHealth's business unit's (Optum) acquisition of DaVita Medical Group in 2019.[3] Although certainly not the only provider/payer strategy in play within the industry, the size of that transaction ($4.3B) made it stand out and markedly increased the awareness of payer partnerships as a driver for affiliation.

Succession Planning. While some executive-level leadership turnover comes as a surprise, in other organizations, there is no designated "heir to the throne." Without the available talent to develop, there may be a complete lack of succession planning until it is too late. It is feasible, however, for an organization to align with another to ensure a pipeline of future leaders.

Provider Recruitment. Recruiting providers can be an emotionally taxing and financially draining endeavor for many organizations. With provider supply low and demand for their talents high, finding a skilled clinician who is also a suitable fit for an organization can be a challenge. Affiliation can assist in this vital work. Through recruitment agreements, particularly those supported by an organization's community needs assessment, organizations can affiliate with providers both during and after they complete their training.

Physician Attrition. As the average age of physicians in the United States continues to rise, an increase in physician retirements looms. The potential for physician attrition through retirement is a reality for many organizations and yet another driving force for affiliation. It becomes essential to bring in new providers faster than the older generation retires, so as not to leave or create access issues.

Nearly every major reason for affiliation is either strategic, operational, financial, or environmental. No one motive or purpose is better or more appropriate than another, and no driver for affiliation guarantees any greater chance of success than any other.

CONCERNS REGARDING AFFILIATION

There are many reasons to affiliate, as documented above, and many reasons not to affiliate. Further, there are reasons affiliations fail. These negative factors should receive equal consideration before a transaction occurs. Due diligence should include consideration of why to and why not to affiliate, as well as reasons an affiliation would succeed and why it could fail.

Benjamin Franklin said, "An ounce of prevention is worth a pound of cure," and this adage still rings true today. Figuring out where the potential potholes in a prospective affiliation lie can be even more important than considering its potential downstream benefits. The reasons not to affiliate and the reasons affiliations fail are discussed more thoroughly below.

Reasons Not to Affiliate

One of the most significant reasons not to affiliate is a desire for better commercial payer reimbursements. Achieving improvements in payer contracts, when the sole or primary motive for affiliation, often proves to be an insufficient reason. Payer contracts can be terminated or renegotiated, and what had been an increase may suddenly erode at the end of the contract term.

Additionally, many payers will make updates to their contracts that disproportionately advantage and/or disadvantage specific codes. In the case of a multi-specialty practice merger, the newly coalesced group may find that their new payer contract increases gastroenterology-specific codes by 20% but reduces urologic-specific codes by 15%. Thus, in this example, although a net gain in rates is achieved, it may not be as beneficial as anticipated because it comes at the cost of harming a part of the group. Without that advantage, organizations may find that there is no longer a reason for unification. If the primary reason for affiliating fizzles and there is no other significant consideration keeping the group together, the entire group may dissolve as well.

Reasons Affiliations Fail

As is discussed in Chapter 17, the act of affiliating seldom is as easy as it seems and often is significantly more difficult than expected. This imbalance between perception and reality causes affiliations to fail. Under-preparedness in operations and relationships is the most common reason affiliations fail. The lack of mental preparation also includes underestimating the complexity of the affiliation process and believing it will be easier than it is.

John Kotter, a best-selling author, Harvard professor and arguably one of the leaders in the area of change management, outlines in his book *Leading Change*, an eight-step process for change. In the fourth step, Kotter calls for a "volunteer army."[4] Much of the operational and relational under-preparedness in healthcare affiliations stems from enlisting an inadequate "volunteer army" to support the change the affiliation demands.

Another reason affiliations fail is improper or inadequate consideration of the legal and regulatory hurdles associated with such relationships. As detailed in Chapter 15, affiliations come with many intricacies, and unless appropriately structured, these complexities can result in noncompliance with applicable regulations. One example is self-referral regulations. When bringing together disparate groups, this area should receive ample consideration by competent counsel.

SUMMARY

Affiliations, which have increased drastically in the healthcare industry over the past three decades and continue to be prevalent, can yield overwhelmingly positive results, including improved quality, increased access, and financial stability. However, careful examination of the reasons for considering affiliation is critical to the enduring success of such affiliation.

This chapter provides numerous factors supporting affiliation, as well as reasons why some affiliations do not stand the test of time. Overall, the most critical reason to affiliate is the one that will benefit your organization the most.

REFERENCES

1. Porter ME. *Competitive Advantage: Creating and Sustaining Superior Performance.* New York: The Free Press; 1985.
2. Shanafelt MD, and Noseworthy JH. Executive Leadership and Physician Well-being: Nine Organizational Strategies to Promote Engagement and Reduce Burnout. *Mayo Clin Proc.* 2017;92(1):129-146. Available at https://www.mayoclinicproceedings.org/article/S0025-6196(16)30625-5/pdf. Accessed September 9, 2019.
3. Coombs B. United Health to Buy DaVita Clinics for $4.9 Billion, CNBC. Wednesday, Dec 6, 2017. https://www.cnbc.com/2017/12/06/unitedhealth-to-buy-davita-clinics-for-4-point-9-billion.html
4. Kotter J. *Leading Change.* Boston: Harvard Business School Press; 1996.

CHAPTER 4

Summary of Current Models

In this chapter, we present more information about the various affiliation models available to physicians, health systems, and other investor/operators, to establish a brief guideline for the consideration of the options "universe."

Using Figure 1.1 from Chapter 1 (page 2) as our primary reference tool, we have an overview of the traditional alignment model descriptions. While there are many variations, this chart provides a summary that applies to every affiliation scenario and will serve as a point of reference throughout this book.

LIMITED, MODERATE, AND FULL INTEGRATION AFFILIATION MODELS

The models, as shown in Figure 1.1, are classified as Limited Integration, Moderate Integration, and Full Integration affiliation models. Following is an explanation of each classification.

Limited Affiliations

Limited affiliation models involve relationships among the relevant parties that stop short of significant long-term integration/affiliation. These models include hospitals and physician groups and encompass such matters as recruitment assistance, medical directorships, and call coverage. The arrangements involve minimal negotiation, and the agreements concern task-oriented relationships.

When the task is complete, the relationship ends until a new mission is defined. Medical directorships, for example, could be task-oriented based on a specific hospital or health system initiative and for a service set for a limited time. Though many medical directorships are for an extended period, the affiliation is limited to the parties involved.

Physicians often consider affiliation with other physicians through *independent practice associations* (IPAs). These loosely formed alliances are designed primarily to aggregate resources for payer contracting; however, unless the IPA is clinically integrated, it may not function as a joint contracting medium. It can align providers on a limited basis without a legal or operational merger.

Other forms of limited affiliation include call coverage agreements and extended contracts such as hospitalists, laborists, and specific services agreements among hospitals and physicians.

Moderate Affiliations

Moderate affiliation models attempt to address more sustaining, ongoing, and lengthier affiliations, although they are not permanent. These arrangements can be effected between physicians and hospitals/health systems through specific agreements to engage the physicians (often specialists) in overall service line management.

For example, orthopedic surgeons would be contracted to help improve the operations and throughput of the operating/surgical services of a hospital. Who better than the physician surgeons to determine best practices and ensure that the efficiencies of surgical services are maximized?

Similar examples of moderate affiliations are service line management and/or clinical co-management. These contractual relationships are often between specific specialties, such as orthopedics, cardiology, and neurosurgery. They not only provide service line management, often tied to the definition and measuring of quality and cost savings, but compensate the physicians based on achievement of established goals and objectives. Co-management agreements are efforts to address the future of value-based reimbursement and accountable care services.

Moderate forms of integration among physician groups include forming management entities such as management services organizations and information systems organizations. These affiliations do not involve merging groups but are efforts to address the opportunities to work together and realize economies of scale, cost savings, and other measures of efficiency.

Joint ventures are moderate affiliation models and can be found among all types of providers/investors. They involve specific initiatives to complete an undertaking, such as shared ownership in a medical office building, surgery center, or other facility. They also can be limited to short duration and address only a specific initiative and expire when completed.

Full Affiliations

Full affiliation involves high levels (and prospectively longer-term or permanent) forms of affiliation. Though there are many such models, employment tends to be the first thought when one considers the definition of full integration. Nevertheless, it is not the only form of total integration, as Figure 1.1 illustrates.

A result of the advent of the Affordable Care Act and the increased focus on value-based medicine and reimbursement is the effort to form CIOs. These entities, while not resulting in merged groups or employment or professional services arrangements among hospitals and physicians, are still examples of full affiliation. For instance, in the most mature clinically integrated network (CIN) structure, physician and hospital constituents are clinically integrated; thus, through care coordination and sharing of clinical data (such as if they merged through a professional services agreement [PSA] or employment agreement) the result is the ability to negotiate contracts jointly. Whether called an accountable care organization (ACO), CIN, or quality collaborative, all apply to a model of full integration.

Employment lite is another form of full integration in that PSAs are structured to mirror many of the characteristics of employment, but they stop short because a contractual relationship exists between the hospitals and healthcare providers (usually physicians). Because of the similarity with employment (e.g., defined terms, compensation parameters, market value and commercially reasonable compensation requirements, incentives tied to performance, and more), PSAs indeed are employment lite and bring about full integration.

Another full affiliation option is for private medical groups to aggregate legally and/or operationally. Regardless of the structure, post-merger, those parties are one single legal entity.

Private equity affiliation is another form of full alignment, but the partner with the physician group is an outside investor, manager, or another party.

VARIATIONS TO THE CORE MODELS

Each of the examples noted above and listed in Figure 1.1 has variations or nuances. For example, PSA models can be structured in four defined ways. These structures are addressed in some detail in Chapter 6. Here, we illustrate that there are variations to the core models and structures. Healthcare managers, consultants, attorneys, and other innovative players are developing new models and will continue along that path as they have over recent years.

One new model, a take-off from private equity transactions, is discussed in Chapter 9. Examples include the *private equity "like"* model and various *joint equity ventures* that can deal with multiple partners/players. These are discussed in Chapter 7.

SPECIAL CONSIDERATIONS

All models require data aggregation and management, regardless of the affiliation plan or its goals and objectives. Chapter 14 addresses the technology considerations in mergers and other forms of affiliation.

Every transaction has legal and regulatory ramifications which require that the structure be considered in light of the legal and regulatory matters, especially between a physician and a hospital, and all other players as well.

Capital procurement is another issue within the affiliation models, meaning that the source of the money is extremely relevant. Investments that are clearly at risk and/or established at arm's length are generally a requirement. Completing pro forma financial analyses and designing the sources of capital are a significant matter, which is addressed in Chapter 16.

SUMMARY

In this chapter, we briefly introduced the possibilities and alternatives for affiliation models. We address these models in more detail in the remaining chapters, along with instances of their viability. These deals and transactions call for expert advisory services from those who understand the processes involved. Chapter 17 summarizes the mechanics for putting together and ultimately closing such varied affiliation models.

While there are numerous models to consider, there are many forms and variations of these structures. We will look at the relevant points for completing a successful affiliation transaction along with an in-depth analysis and the structural considerations for each prototype as we get into the details of each model. No matter the relationship of the affiliates (i.e., physicians, multi- or single-specialty groups, hospitals/health systems, private equity, management companies, ancillary entities, or another), the needs of a well-planned and firmly developed structure make it imperative to reach a win-win scenario for all the players.

CHAPTER 5

Physician Employment

With the options for affiliation addressed previously, this chapter provides an in-depth review of physician employment. This discussion will cover the structure and reality of employment along with the economic impact of employment through compensation. We will address the most common items relating to employment with the understanding that each situation is unique and can vary over time.

EXAMINING EMPLOYMENT

Employed vs. Self-Employed

A recent study by the American Medical Association (AMA) revealed that employed physicians outnumber those who are self-employed for the first time in United States history. The AMA Physician Practice Benchmark Survey report states, "Employed physicians were 47.4% of all patient care physicians in 2018, up 6% since 2012. In contrast, self-employed physicians were 45.9% of all patient care physicians in 2018, down 7% since 2012."[1]

Although these data represent a large shift in the marketplace, the trend is nothing new. In the 1990s, for instance, the percentage of self-employed physicians decreased drastically and rapidly. While numerous factors can play a part in the shift to employment, it is a combination of a few key components that is affecting physicians today.

As healthcare evolves to keep pace with progressive technology, electronic health records (EHRs) have become a staple of modern-day medical practice. The transition from paper charts to EHRs, however, requires considerable capital investment and obliges the physicians to change their practice patterns and learn something new. Also, along with technological advancements comes the need for data collection and reporting. The sheer volume of potential data available is overwhelming, and this vast amount of information must be translated and reported into meaningful results.

Healthcare has the spotlight of both consumers and federal and state governments due to the growth and dollars associated with the marketplace. To curb healthcare spending and costs, regulations and mandates have emerged that make navigating the patient care continuum more tedious and detailed. Both government payers and private payers are moving more dollars to be "at-risk" to offset the rising costs of care, which has garnered substantial public attention.

The shift from fee-for-services to fee-for-value payment structures has led to legislation like the Medicare Access and CHIP Reauthorization Act of 2015 (MACRA), commercial risk-models, and state-based initiatives centered around the reported data and patient cost management. With both carrot and stick models in place, more risk has shifted to physicians over the past 5–10 years.

Additionally, physicians have shifted to employment due to a higher priority on healthier work/life balance than those before them. Employment provides physicians with a level of personal security, which simultaneously allows them to explore other areas of the medical field through administrative duties.

A combination of these key factors has driven the increase in physician employment. As the marketplace forces more risk and responsibility on physicians, they will continue to find employment as the most attractive affiliation model.

Realities of Employment

Of the various alignment options from which physicians can choose, employment is the highest form of integration, because the employer assumes responsibility for many of the business and operational functions. Of course, there are different structures to employment, and carve-outs can always be negotiated. Figures 5.1, 5.2, and 5.3 illustrate three types of employment structures.

Figure 5.1 shows a Group Without Walls structure in which the organization is set up as a separate management entity to run the provider business operations.

Figure 5.2 shows a Group Practice Subsidiary. Physicians can be part of the employment model while still retaining some autonomy. A few physicians sit on the board as ultimate decision makers, although other physicians can contribute through committees focused on topics like

FIGURE 5.1. Group Without Walls ("GWW")

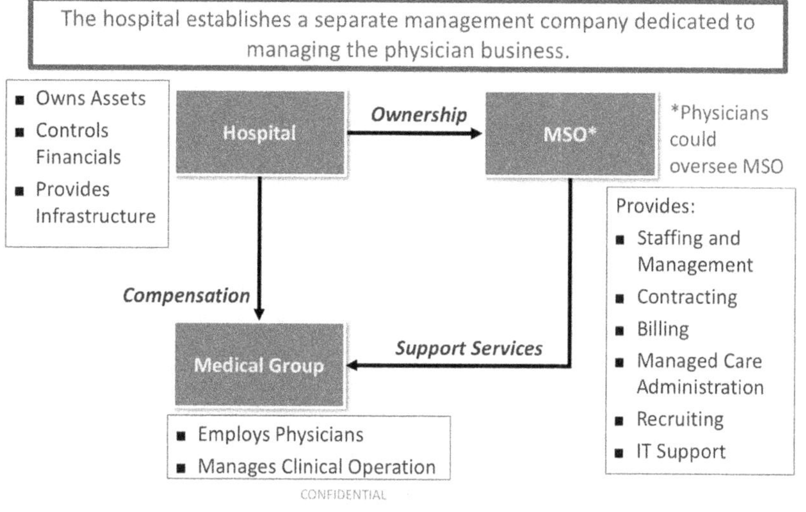

FIGURE 5.2. Group Practice Subsidiary ("GPS")

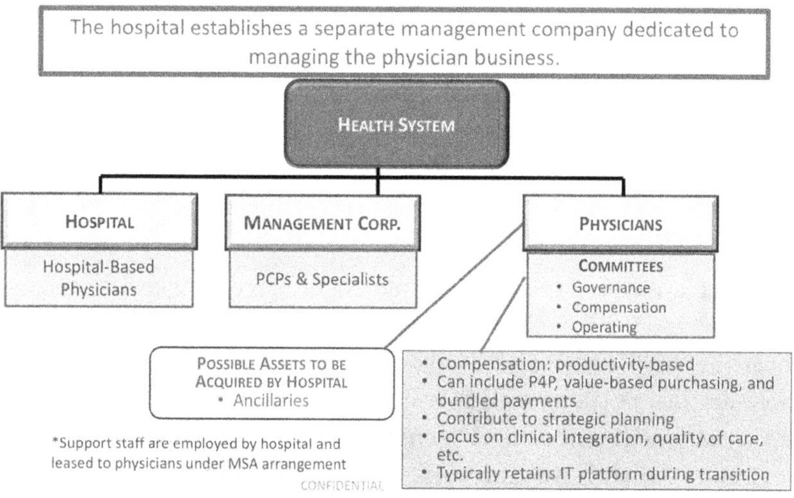

finance or operations. Also, the medical group takes charge of the clinical administrative duties, allowing the employed physicians to operate as if they were self-employed.

Figure 5.3 represents an illustration of a Dyad Model. This model separates the employed providers by service focus (e.g., pediatric spe-

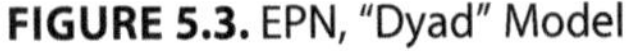
FIGURE 5.3. EPN, "Dyad" Model

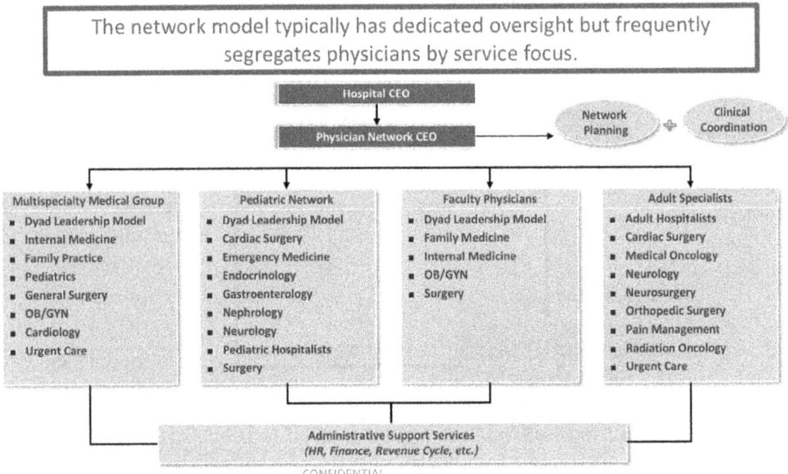

cialties, faculty physicians, adult surgical specialties, etc.) with each service focus having dyad leadership.

In these figures, the hospital is responsible for most of the administrative support (billing and collecting, human resources, revenue cycle, etc.) as well as the compensation terms. The physician remains responsible for the clinical services provided.

Employment Agreements

Let's take a deeper look at an employment agreement to understand what it means to be an employed physician. The following explanations cover the high-level basics like compensation, as well as some of the more detailed portions such as restrictive covenants. They are some of the common elements found in employment agreements.

- **Hospital staff membership.** Physician must maintain membership in good standing on the active medical staff during the term of the agreement. Physician will comply with all rules and regulations of the medical staff as defined in the medical staff bylaws.
- **Clinical services.** Defines the full-time equivalent (FTE) for the clinical services provided and the exceptions to the stated FTE. Section states the medical specialty in which the physicians will provide professional medical services.

- **Term.** Length of agreement between physician and employer, with standard term lengths lasting three years or five years. Term section generally includes automatic renewal term length. (Long-term agreements, such as three- and five-year terms, were once standard and are still common, but many healthcare organizations and practices are moving toward one-year agreements.)
- **Termination.** Termination without cause requires prior written notice of XX number of days (most common are 90 days, 120 days, and 180 days). Termination sections also include the for-cause termination clauses.
- **Compensation.** Consists of standard language without details of economics; these usually are in an addendum/exhibit. The compensation addendum/exhibit defines the compensation terms and the corresponding economics for each term. Professional expense amounts and compensation caps are defined in this section, as needed.
- **Benefits.** General benefit language is used in the body of the agreement, and the details of the benefits are provided in an exhibit. Benefits generally include retirement, health insurance, disability insurance, life insurance, time off, etc. Benefits are specifically defined in the agreement or referred to in the organization's benefit plans/policies.
- **Professional Liability Insurance.** Employer will pay for and/or maintain professional liability insurance in amounts no less than as may be required pursuant to medical staff bylaws. The policy will provide coverage for the services rendered by the physician. Employers also provide extended professional liability insurance (also known as tail coverage) which covers acts, errors, or omissions of professional negligence occurring within the scope of employment once the agreement has been terminated or expired.
- **Support Staff.** Employer will incur all applicable expenses relating to staffing (including professional, non-professional, clerical, paramedical, and nursing personnel) for the proper function for all clinical services rendered by the physician.
- **Space, Equipment, Supplies.** Employer will provide and pay for office space necessary for performance of the services in the agreement. Employer will also provide and repair all equipment and supplies as needed.

- **Billing and Collections.** Employer will be responsible for billing patients and third-party payers for services performed by physician and will collect the fees for such services.
- **Outside activities.** Physician will not, without prior written consent, engage in or participate in any venture or activity that the employer may consider to be competitive with, or adverse to, the business of the employer. Additionally, work belonging to the employer includes all work contributed to, created by, or to be created by physician in the course of performing obligations under the agreement.
- **Restrictive Covenants.** Includes the restricted entities and restricted territory the physicians cannot interact with/in for a defined period (generally one to two years). The restricted entities are direct competitors of the employer, and the restricted territory is commonly a 15-mile radius from the locations in which the physician-provided services. Employers define and detail their confidential information to be kept by physician in the restrictive covenants section.
- **Additional duties.** Duties not explicitly defined and explained within the agreement are noted in detail in this section. The additional duties can be requirements of the physician as part of the employment or can include duties to be performed in addition to the defined services.

The employment agreement is the structure for all physician-provided services. Creating employment agreements with clear, well-defined terms is an important part of a functioning relationship between providers and administration. Legal counsel (the draftee of the employment agreements) should aim for all terms to be consistent, where applicable, and understandable by all parties. Ambiguity within an employment agreement can generate confusion regarding the services and responsibilities of the provider, tension between providers and administration, and in worst-case scenarios, legal action by one of the parties.

Compensation Within Employment

When contemplating employment, a crucial consideration for physicians is personal compensation. For the employer, physician compensation is one of the most significant expense items within their physician network. Thus, finding the right balance so physicians are satisfied and the employer is financially responsible makes compensation a central piece in physician employment. As the details of employment compensation are discussed, it is helpful to have a macro idea as to key considerations that impact physician compensation in today's market. Figure 5.4 illustrates the three macro considerations that must be kept in mind.

FIGURE 5.4. Macro Considerations in Employment Compensation

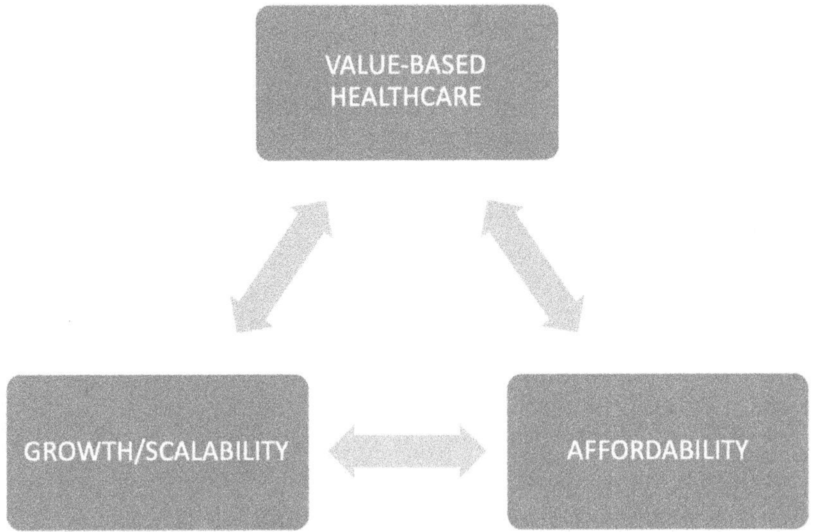

- **Value-Based Healthcare:** The industry has shifted toward a focus on the quality of care instead of volume. Risk is shifting to the providers with an emphasis on care management, cost reduction, and prevention. The shift is due to increased scrutiny on the industry with the quality of care provided not equating to the number of dollars spent on care.
- **Affordability:** The market shift to value-based care and the corresponding risk shifted to physicians has increased the cost burden on physicians. In an employment setting, physicians can provide services in the new environment without the additional concern for financial feasibility.

- **Growth/Scalability:** Moving to employment gives physicians the security they desire while also allowing the hospital/system to grow their services. A compensation policy aligned with the strategic goals of the organization offers a model capable of scaling as the organization grows.

Strategic Review

Whether designing a compensation model for a single physician or redesigning a compensation structure for an entire group of physicians, the first step in designing a compensation plan/model is performing a strategic review of historical compensation and related factors. Strategic review is divided into three phases: review of historical data, qualitative review, and analysis.

Phase one, review of historical data, is as literal as it sounds. Those developing the compensation plan should review all productivity, compensation, and compensation calculations. Understanding the historical compensation components allows for the proposed compensation plan to be adjusted in areas where changes may be needed without complete disruption to physician compensation. Along with the historical data, the most recent community needs assessment should be reviewed to gain greater insight into the depth of the supply and demand for each specialty within the market.

Phase two in the strategic review is a qualitative review. Although less data-driven, this phase is nonetheless important for understanding the impact of compensation and compensation modeling. Discussions with key stakeholders will provide the employer and physicians a better understanding of the current landscape. Those who have input on the compensation design should educate themselves about the local and national market for any specialty being contemplated as part of a redesign.

Once the due diligence for phases one and two is complete, the current model and potential changes to the model should be analyzed in conjunction with the goals of the organization. The compensation model design should align with the employer's goals, and the organization can begin the detailed designing of the compensation model via model variables.

Model Variables

In most hospital-employed compensation models, the three primary components that generate a compensation model are the target rate per wRVU, base pay, and the base wRVU threshold. (Note: A relative value unit [RVU] describes a unit of work for each CPT™® code billed within that organized system of structure. For each CPT code, there are three components of services rendered and assigned an RVU value. These values are then summed to create the RVU for that specific code. The three components are the work-only component [wRVU], the practice expense component [PE RVU], and the professional liability insurance [MP RVU]. Reimbursement for Medicare is derived by multiplying the total RVU value by the then-current assigned conversion factor.) Certain specialties, such as radiology, hospitalists, and other hospital-based specialties, have different models that do not focus on the three components. To create a model that is both simple and functional, priority should be given to setting the model variables within the target rate per wRVU; then base pay and the base wRVU threshold can be addressed.

Target Rate per wRVU

The organization should determine the method to be used in setting the target rate per wRVU. Two key methods for setting the target rate are using market data and historical/projected collections per wRVU. Figure 5.5 details the pros and cons of each method. Every organization will need to determine the appropriate balance between the methods that best fit them based on the information learned during their strategic review. The goal of using these methods is to set a rate that is market-based and financially viable for the organization.

FIGURE 5.5. Methods for Setting Target Rate

Market Data		Collections per wRVU	
Pros	**Cons**	**Pros**	**Cons**
Represents the national market	May not be financially sustainable	Represents actual financial scenario	May not represent market recruiting rates
Same rate (as a %ile) set for all specialties	Assumes all specialties should be at the same rate (as a %ile)	Rates will reflect specialty-specific financial performance	Difficult to set specialty rates if provider performance varies greatly
Updates every year	Updates may not reflect local market changes	Data are current and reflect current market	Local market changes have big impact

Ultimately, the target rate should be market-based, as that amount will be needed to recruit/retain; however, it also should be financially viable. Both fair market value (FMV) and financial viability should limit what you can (FMV) and should (financial viability) pay. While it is in no way an indication of FMV, compensation and productivity tend to be in alignment when using a target rate near the median of market data. This relationship breaks down as the rate deviates from the median. Should the target rate be set below the median, productivity likely will outpace compensation; compensation will outpace productivity if the target rate is above the median.

At this point the organization has determined the method for setting the target rate and the market percentile the target rate should hit. A top-down approach is preferred to generate the fully loaded target rate per wRVU, which includes multiple forms of compensation (productivity, performance, other). As shown in Figure 5.6, the top-down approach achieves the target rate per wRVU, while the bottom-up approach makes it more difficult to control the economics of the model over time.

FIGURE 5.6. Top-Down vs. Bottom-Up Approaches

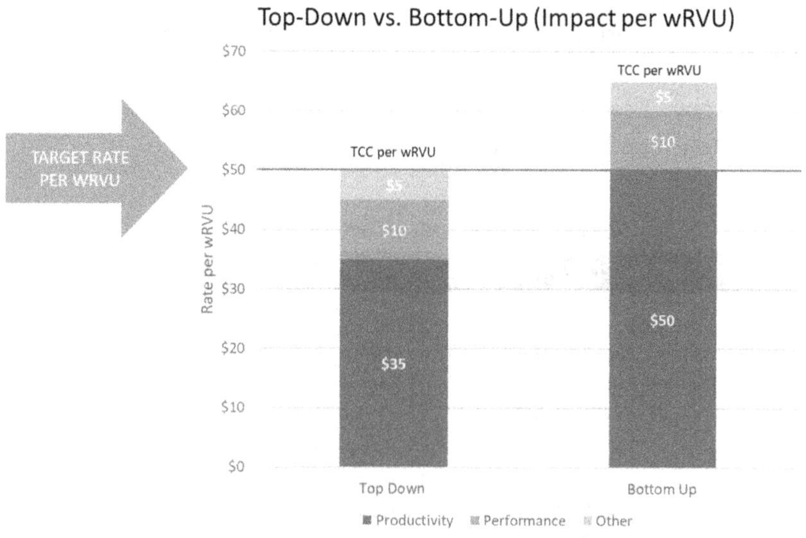

The components that add up to the target rate per wRVU, such as productivity, performance, and other components, must now be allocated. Only by achieving maximum performance for all three components can the full value of the target rate be earned. Generally, allocation among the components is 75%–85% wRVU productivity, 10%–20% individual/group performance incentive, and 5% other components. Primary care is more aggressive with the allocation toward performance incentive (15%–20%) since the metrics and ability to track the metrics are more developed. On the other hand, specialty care has not gone as far with performance incentive weighting. Unless organizations have been tracking performance metrics for a time, specialty care allocates 5%–10% of compensation to performance incentive.

Other High-Level Components

Before examining the details of the target rate per wRVU components, the other two high-level components of the compensation model should be addressed: base pay and wRVU threshold. Base pay should be established based on what best aligns with the overarching goals of the organization and maintains physicians' attitude toward their compensation. The base wRVU threshold is a product of the target rate per wRVU and established base pay since the threshold will be calculated via dividing the base pay by the target rate per wRVU.

Base Compensation Structure

Establishing base compensation is a significant part of the employed physician model. Base compensation allows for consistent compensation pay period to pay period. In establishing base compensation, it is critical to remember that *the goal of base compensation is to ensure consistency in pay without compromising the incentive structure of the model.* There are three preferred methods of base compensation to support the compensation modeling: base draw, guarantee, and hybrid guarantee. All three methods have their pros and cons; thus, an organization must decide which one is right for each situation.

1. **Base Draw.** A base draw is non-guaranteed compensation based on historical total cash compensation. To ensure the level of the draw is appropriate, all components of compensation should be considered and not focused solely on productivity compensation. Many base draw models err on the side of being over conservative by having the base draw set at a percentage of the previous year's total compensation—for example, 85%–90% of total compensa-

tion. Base draw presents a risk for the physician in that should productivity and performance not achieve historical levels, the physician may owe back compensation paid if the compensation was not earned.

2. **Guarantee.** Since guarantees place risk only on the organization, fully guaranteed base compensation should be applied only to new physicians during a two- to three-year ramp-up period. Long-term guarantees can bring risk of misalignment between compensation and productivity, with an inequity of cost-to-collections being economically unsustainable. However, there are instances when long-term guarantees can be appropriate. In less desirable and rural markets, a long-term guarantee may be the only way to recruit physicians to an organization. Rural markets frequently face this issue because the market does not have the volume to sustain the physician.
3. **Hybrid Guarantee.** In markets that need longer-term base guarantees, a hybrid guarantee base compensation model can be a useful strategy for applying some conservatism to a model. Base compensation would stay the same only if productivity is within XX% of supporting the base pay. Base pay cannot be adjusted more than XX% per year. Figure 5.7 provides an example of a hybrid guarantee.

The hybrid model changes base compensation only in the upcoming year. Incentive compensation is not affected within a current year if the physician is on pace to be outside of the corridor. For example, in the illustration, Physician C would receive the full amount of productivity compensation earned based on productivity exceeding the threshold, and in the next year the threshold for Physician C would change.

Productivity Incentive

With the three high-level components being addressed, let's consider the component of the target rate per wRVU. The largest portion of the target rate is the productivity incentive. The driver for the productivity incentive is a physician's wRVUs, which are the norm for measuring productivity in today's market. The most current Medicare Physician Fee Schedule should be used to calculate wRVUs, inclusive of modifiers. Calculating the physician compensation based on productivity

FIGURE 5.7. Hybrid Guarantee—
10% Productivity Corridor Illustration

	A	B	C
Base wRVU Threshold	5,000	5,000	5,000
Actual wRVUs	4,000	5,250	7,000
Percent Difference	-20%	5%	40%
Base Compensation	$200,000	$200,000	$200,000
Adjustment to Base Comp	-10%	0%	10%
Adjusted Base Comp	$180,000	$200,000	$220,000

Example

- Physician A generates 4,000 wRVUs
  —Productivity is more than 10% below the base threshold
  —Base compensation is reduced 10%
- Physician B generates 5,000 wRVUs
  —Productivity is within the 10% productivity corridor
  —Base compensation remains the same
- Physician C generates 7,000 wRVUs
  —Productivity is more than 10% above the base threshold
  —Base compensation is only increased 10%

should be on the same schedule for all physicians (quarterly, semi-annually, annually). Productivity compensation models range in complexity with the most common models being single-tier and two-tier. A single-tier model pays all wRVUs at a single rate (dollar amount). Two-tier models pay one rate up to a certain number of wRVUs and pay a different rate for all wRVUs above the tier threshold. A single-tier model is recommended for the productivity incentive as this model is the simplest and easiest to administer.

Performance Incentive

A performance incentive does not have the same value tied to it as a productivity incentive; however, the value and emphasis placed on performance have grown over the past decade and the marketplace continues to shift more focus on performance.

To build a performance incentive, the organization must first determine what it wants to incentivize. There should be an appropriate balance between the value of the incentive and associated metrics, which is best achieved through collaboration between administration and physicians. The organization should choose metrics that align with their goals but should also allow the physicians to choose some metrics. They should only be paid out semi-annually or annually through an objective scoring mechanism to ensure the chosen metrics are properly tracked and accounted. Additionally, the performance incentive can incorporate individual and group performance. The structure of individual and group incentives is detailed in Figure 5.8. The figure also provides an example of how to manage each incentive.

FIGURE 5.8. Structure of Individual and Group Incentives

INDIVIDUAL INCENTIVE

- Scorecard based approach
- Not an all or nothing incentive
- The quality committee should decide each year which metrics are most relevant
- Paid out annually based on achievement of individual goals
- Suggested categories:
  —Quality
  —Patient Satisfaction
  —Expense Control
  —Citizenship/Peer Review
  —Access

GROUP INCENTIVE

- Organization-wide goals or measures
- Goals that require a team effort to achieve
- Reward providers for exceptional group performance
- Opportunity of 5% of the target rate for all specialties
- Paid out annually based on achievement of group goals
- Suggested categories:
  —Organizational stretch goals
  —Quality
  —Financial performance

Panel Incentive

Panel incentive is an example of another component of the target rate per wRVU. Panel incentive, for primary care providers, is a way to incentivize access, recognize non-wRVU-generating activities, and shift the provider mindset toward capitation.

Two primary methods for calculating panel are EHR-defined and manual calculation. The EHR-defined calculation comes from the EHR system based on rendering provider. Because organizations allow the rendering provider field to be fully editable by staff, a provider's actual panel can vary from the EHR-defined calculation. Manual calculation uses an historical review report to determine who is the primary provider for a patient. Here are three forms of panel incentives with varying impact on the compensation model:

FIGURE 5.9. Using Panel Size to Determine Specific Performance Incentive

Method II

Illustration	Total	Note
Total Primary Care wRVUs	122,550	A
Panel Incentive (per wRVU) Weight	$4.08	B
Total Panel Incentive Pool	**$500,004**	A x B = C
Total Primary Care Panel	50,000	D
Per Member Rate	**$10.00**	C / D = E
Individual Physician Panel Size	2,000	F (per MD)
Panel Incentive Opportunity	**$20,000**	G = E x F
Quality Performance Score (Results)	75%	H
Panel Incentive Compensation	**$15,000**	I = G x H

- The least impact panel incentive is establishing a per-member, per-month/per-member, per-year compensation value and multiplying by a physician's panel size. This recognizes access, team-based care, and required work that is not wRVU-generating. The value associated with this method should be meaningful but not more significant than that.
- A slightly more impactful method for using panel incentives is using panel size to determine the specific performance incentive opportunity. Actual payment of performance incentives is predicated on achievement of established metrics. This method connects panel incentive to performance incentive, causing the physician to focus on managing a specific population's health. Figure 5.9 illustrates this method.
- The third and most economically influential method involving panel entails shifting fully from productivity incentive to panel incentive as most of the physician compensation. Figure 5.10 illustrates an example of using panel incentive as the driver of most of the physician compensation.

All the model variables included in an employed compensation model combine to account for total cash compensation (TCC). It is important for TCC to make economic sense from both an organizational perspective and a market data perspective, but the individual

FIGURE 5.10. Using Panel as the Driver of Compensation

Method III

Illustration	Total	Note
Physician Panel Size	2,000	A
Panel Incentive Weight - PMPM	$10.00	B
Total Panel Incentive Pool	**$20,000**	A x B = C
Months in Year	12	D
Total Cash Compensation - Annual	**$240,000**	C x D = E
Base Compensation Allocation @ 90%	$216,000	F
Panel Incentive Allocation @ 10%	**$24,000**	G
Quality Performance Score (Results)	75%	H
Panel Incentive Compensation	**$18,000**	I = G x H
Total Cash Compensation (Paid)	**$234,000**	J = F + I

model components should also make economic sense. Compensation should be viewed as both a sum of the components, TCC, and individual components. Thus, there is a need to monitor TCC economically and structurally.

Governance

Governance of compensation is a three-pronged approach that consists of a compensation committee, compensation policy, and compensation plan. The compensation committee is in place to govern the issues and structures of compensation. The committee is often a subset of the medical group board and would be structures as illustrated in Figure 5.11.

An established compensation policy focuses the attention of all stakeholders on key tenets of the compensation structure. Policy is a vehicle to ensure the compensation structure adheres to the mission/vision/values of the organization. It will outline policies and procedures with respect to FMV and commercial reasonableness by addressing some of the questions that follow:

- What triggers an internal review?
- What is sent out for external review?

FIGURE 5.11. Governance Committee Structure

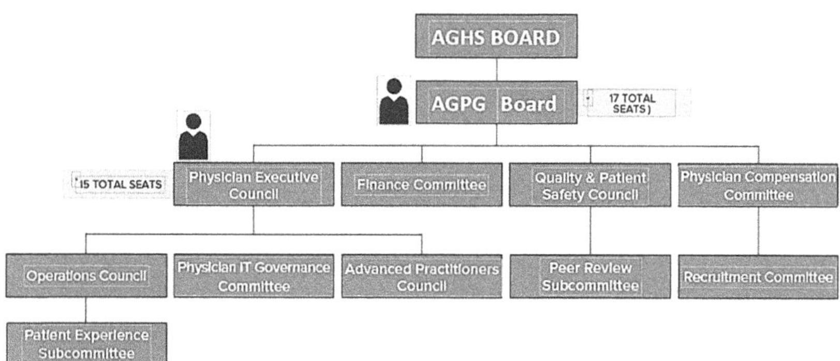

- How to adjudicate issues to the extent they exist?
- How often should FMV reviews be performed for all employed physician?

A compensation model document should include a compensation policy. This document will ensure terms are consistent across all physicians/specialties, outline key tenets of compensation structure outside of employment agreement, allow for simplicity in updating model, illustrate key components of structure, and document crucial terms.

SUMMARY

The highest form of affiliation is employment. Within the current healthcare landscape, value-based healthcare, affordability, and growth/scalability are the central focus for physicians and administrators to ensure successful employment models. Other forms of alignment and integration are available for entities and physicians based on what is right for their situation. It happens, however, that employment is trending to be the popular choice in the current market.

CHAPTER 6

Professional Services Agreements

Historically, health systems viewed employment as the best option to meet community needs, especially in more rural areas where recruitment is often difficult. The physicians were an essential part of the revenue stream under a volume-based model. As the healthcare landscape transforms, health systems are beginning to see the benefits of partnering with physicians outside of employment, so long as the arrangements are economically sound and substantiated.

From the practice's or physician's perspective, alignment with a health system is attractive because of the stability it provides from an operational standpoint. This allows private practice physicians to focus on the clinical aspects of care rather than on the business functions.

Even though private practices and health systems realize that alignment is necessary and beneficial, many practices want to maintain their ownership and are reluctant to dive headfirst into an employment arrangement with a health system. In this chapter, we will discuss one level of integration, a professional services agreement (PSA).

A PSA is a favorite alignment model used to form stronger partnerships between privately owned practices and health systems without engaging in a full-employment arrangement. Many private practices seek to maintain stability and independence while also receiving financial and operational support from a health system. We call this type of arrangement "employment lite."

TYPES OF PSAs

A PSA arrangement between a physician practice and a health system typically falls into one of four basic models:

1. Global Payment PSA

2. Practice Management Arrangement (PMA)
3. Traditional PSA
4. Carve-Out PSA

While these models are foundational and are the most common models, each can be modified in countless ways to meet the needs of the organization. The many variations of each model allow the potentially aligning organizations to mix and match the desired qualities of each within their PSA structure. This hybrid approach can become a factor as negotiations unfold, particularly as second-generation agreements are renegotiated. Nevertheless, the general terms of PSAs likely will have the core key tenets to serve as a starting point for discussions and negotiations between the organizations to finalize an agreement that meets everyone's needs and goals.

Global Payment PSA

The global payment PSA model most closely resembles the practice as it was before alignment. Specifically, physicians and staff remain employed by the practice, and practice management remains at its pre-PSA structure. The practice is contracted to provide professional services to the health system or other entity, and that entity now owns the revenue stream for those professional services. The health system is responsible for payer contract negotiations, billing, collections, and the entire revenue cycle. The physicians and all support staff remain employed by the practice and receive compensation and benefits from the practice.

The practice receives payment for services based on the terms and conditions defined by the PSA documentation. The payment terms typically are productivity based (usually using wRVUs), along with potential non-productivity-based incentives. Payment per wRVU is the most popular and easy-to-construct model for determining compensation; however, as reimbursement continues to shift toward value-based and performance-based fees, the compensation structure for physicians is also changing.

Now, compensation is also tied to something beyond simply production. For example, some agreements currently place a portion of total compensation at risk for value-based tenets. (Note: A relative value unit [RVU] describes a unit of work for each CPT™® code billed within that organized system of structure. For each CPT code, there are three components of services rendered and assigned an RVU value. These values are then summed to create the RVU for that specific code. The three components are the work-only component [wRVU], the practice expense component [PE RVU], and the professional liability insurance [MP RVU]. Reimbursement for Medicare is derived by multiplying the total RVU value by the then-current assigned conversion factor.)

In addition to production-based compensation, the practice receives remuneration for its overhead, typically on a budgeted dollar basis. This budgeted amount reimburses the practice for most of its overhead on a fixed or budgeted basis. It is common to see reimbursement for variable expenses based on a rate per wRVU, as these expenses typically vary with revenue (e.g., drug or medical supplies).

Alternately, the practice may be reimbursed using a total rate per wRVU, although this is becoming less common, as arrangements based on a budgeted overhead reimbursement basis typically are preferred. Figure 6.1 illustrates the potential payment methods discussed under a global payment PSA, with Option 1 being the most prevalent of the two.

FIGURE 6.1. Payment Alternatives Within the Global Payment PSA Model

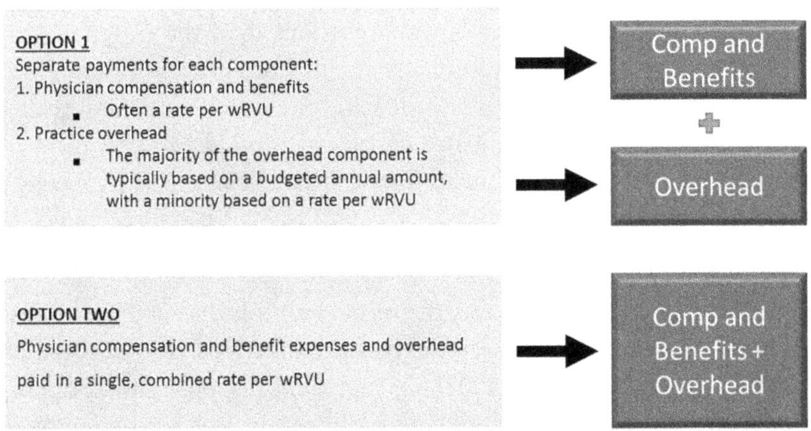

In summary, the global payment PSA is a logical arrangement between a hospital and a practice, offering the practice the customary independence and autonomy, while functioning as a prospective segue

toward full alignment in the future. The global payment PSA provides a positive means of initiating and maintaining a working relationship between two parties.

Practice Management Arrangement

Unlike the other PSA models, under the PMA structure, the physicians and advanced practice providers (APPs), if applicable, are employed by the hospital. The infrastructure of the practice remains independent, and the management and administration continue to support the now-employed providers. One fundamental tenet of the model is that keeping the practice infrastructure makes it easier to transition back to private practice if a long-term arrangement ends. Alternatively, it can easily be transferred to the full ownership of the hospital.

Under the PMA model, the physicians operate as managers of the practice, which now functions more like a back-office support structure, providing administrative services, space, equipment, and support staff. The hospital contracts with the practice for these support services through a fair market value (FMV) management fee. Compensation for the physicians and APPs is consistent with other W-2 employed providers at the health system.

The PMA model typically used when the physicians already have a management services organization (MSO) in place, or they believe their management structure is more efficient than the hospital with which they are aligning. Additionally, the practice may be hesitant that the alignment with the hospital will stand the test of time and need a structure to allow for confidence and trust to build between the two entities. Figure 6.2, below, illustrates the structure of the PMA model.

Traditional PSA

The traditional PSA is arguably the most common PSA and the closest to full employment in the way the practice functions. The hospital or other entity assumes all practice management responsibilities, operational and administrative duties, and all support staff and employees of the practice transition to employment by the hospital. The practice entity remains intact, and the physicians (and potentially APPs) remain employees of the practice. The practice contracts with the hospital for professional services provided by the physicians and APPs.

FIGURE 6.2. Practice Management Arrangement Model

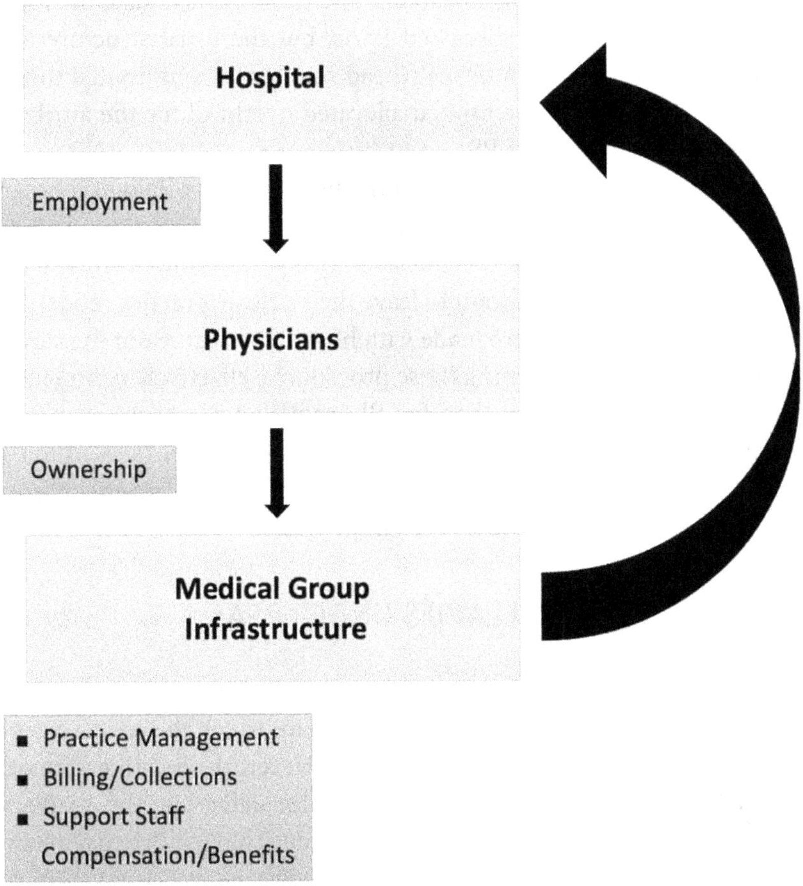

Hospital

Employment

Physicians

Ownership

Medical Group Infrastructure

- Practice Management
- Billing/Collections
- Support Staff Compensation/Benefits

Operationally, the ultimate result resembles employment in that the practice transitions all *ownership* of management and operations to the hospital and is no longer directly responsible for these functions. This transfer relieves the practice of the economic risk of operating a practice and allows the physicians to focus solely on providing quality clinical care to patients. While many physicians see this shift as a positive, others view this type of structure as a loss of control.

Carve-Out PSAs

The carve-out PSA is unique in that it involves a subset of the practice aligning with a strategic partner rather than the entire practice engaging in a PSA. This occurs when a single specialty within a private multispecialty group aligns with a hospital. The carve-out can take the form of any of the previously discussed PSAs, but the usual structure is a global payment PSA, with the overhead reimbursement limited to the direct overhead and some limited allocated overhead for the attributable physicians within the PSA.

This type of arrangement gained traction when cardiologists began realizing significant cuts in reimbursement for echo and nuclear studies. Many physicians sought stability in the reimbursement for these services but did not want to leave their private practice model. As a result, arrangements were made with hospitals to carve out the cardiologists who were performing those procedures, effectively contracting for specific services rather than for all professional services provided. Hospitals continue to use this model to contract with physicians to fill particular needs that do not necessarily require an entire practice or even a total full-time equivalent (FTE) provider.

ANCILLARIES UNDER PSAs

The assumption of ancillary services are negotiable terms in the various PSA models. The practice entity does not have to sell the ancillary services but may retain them if so desired; however, the health system or hospital entity usually takes responsibility for delivering the ancillary services and attaining the subsequent revenue. The practice may retain ownership of the assets that support the ancillaries and lease them to the hospital or sell them outright. Either way, the revenue stream of income shifts to the health system.

ADDITIONAL SERVICES WRAPAROUNDS

In addition to the four main PSA models discussed above, there may be opportunities available to the physicians or hospital that are above and beyond the baseline scope of the services defined within the PSA. These are called wraparound services and are generally wrapped into the core PSA model. The most common wraparound services are:

- Clinical co-management
- Shared cost savings initiatives

- Administrative duties
- APP supervisory duties
- Teaching functions
- Research
- Medical directorships
- Call responsibilities

Most of these wraparounds are *in addition* to the professional services provided by the practice within a PSA model and are compensated in addition to what is defined within the PSA terms for professional services, assuming that the compensation is legitimately earned and within FMV limitations, and the work completed is appropriately documented by the physician. One caveat is that physicians must be willing to forego clinical responsibilities to perform these duties, as they cannot be completed and compensated simultaneously.

Another wraparound that is becoming more common in PSA relationships is an incentive for quality. As discussed previously, the reimbursement for professional services is shifting from volume to value, and with that comes reimbursement for reported quality outcomes. In its most basic form, an incentive payment to physicians for reporting on actual cost, quality, and/or outcome data is applied. Alternatively, PSA models can include at-risk compensation to physicians for demonstrating achievement of both high-quality and cost-efficient care. In some instances, shared savings programs are implemented based on the improvement of quality scores and the reduction in penalties from the Centers for Medicare and Medicaid Services (CMS). Wraparound scenarios offer opportunities for additional forms of alignment, in a limited fashion, and complement the core PSA structure.

LEGAL CHALLENGES

Many of the same legal considerations that apply to employment arrangements apply to the PSA models. It is essential that all parties involved are aware of these issues to ensure that they stay within the confines of the law.

Specifically, the issues of FMV and commercial reasonableness of compensation rates are present in any PSA model, as well as in wraparound agreements. Additionally, the hospital or health system must certify that the PSA does not violate Stark Law through referrals of patients or any federal Anti-Kickback statutes. While these two points cover most federal regulatory issues, the hospital still must be educated and aware of any state laws that may impose even stricter restrictions on PSA arrangements.

OVERALL BENEFITS OF PSA MODELS

There are advantages and disadvantages to the PSA model. We consider these aspects in this section.

Disadvantages

The disadvantages are limited in number and can be easily negotiated by the parties to ensure satisfaction across the board regarding the structure of the PSA. The disadvantages of a PSA include:

- A PSA provides the practice and physicians less stability than employment.
- PSAs are more complex arrangements than employment.
- The inclusion of a non-compete or exclusivity provision is less desirable to some physicians.

Hospitals may be ill-equipped to manage private practices.

While these matters may be deal breakers for some practices contemplating an alignment structure, these points can all be addressed through productive discussions and negotiations between the parties.

Advantages

The benefits of PSAs include:

- The practice maintains independence and autonomy.
- PSAs are more complex arrangements but offer high flexibility for the physicians.
- Physicians keep practice benefit plans in place.
- Support staff may be employed by the hospital and receive better benefit plans.
- PSA structures can segue into full employment or participation in the hospital's clinically integrated network (CIN) or accountable care organization (ACO).

- Hospitals can support complex reimbursement trends due to a more robust infrastructure.
- PSAs offer opportunities to increase revenue and control costs.
- Physicians and hospitals can expand services together without being fully aligned.
- Disengagement/unwind is typically easier than with employment and will enable physicians to return to private practice or partner with someone else.

Clearly, one of the most popular advantages of PSA arrangements is the ability to maintain some level of independence as a practice.

REIMBURSEMENT TRENDS AND PSAs

As reimbursement trends continue the shift from volume to value, many private practices are realizing that their models are a more cost-effective solution than are hospital-owned entities, and they allow them to maintain control of the decision making of their practices. Health systems seek to align with supportive and engaging physicians to drive value through quality care and outcomes. These desires on both sides provide a unique opportunity to work together to meet each other's needs. The private practice physicians can drive value from the front lines through the leadership of quality and outcomes-based initiatives, while the hospital provides a full spectrum of financial and operational resources to allow the practice to be successful.

As value-based care and the related reimbursement trends continue to move forward, health systems and private practices alike will lean on each other to balance the economic pressures, including regulatory demands, administrative and infrastructure needs, decreasing reimbursement rates, and ongoing business operations, all while improving the quality of patient care to be successful in this new paradigm.

IS A PSA RIGHT FOR YOU?

Figure 6.3 provides a questionnaire that can be used to evaluate whether pursuing a PSA model is appropriate and to help determine the best alignment model opportunity for either a hospital/health

FIGURE 6.3. PSA Questionnaire

Question	Answer
1. What does the practice prefer regarding overall structure relative to its alignment? For example, does the practice believe that the hospital's management structure is lacking? Are there questions in the minds of the practice about the sustainability of the hospital management structure? Does the hospital currently provide adequate support services for its aligned practices?	
2. Is there a strong preference among the parties (both the practice and the hospital/health system) for the staff to be employees?	
3. What is the gestalt of the parties relative to ancillary services? What applicable state and federal legal requirements and parameters surround the issue? Is it essential for the hospital/health system to own the ancillary services going forward?	
4. How are leadership and governance addressed? What voting rights and reserved powers may the health system require? What will be the effect of ethical and religious directives, if applicable?	
5. What value-based criteria are to be considered and how will they affect the PSA model going forward? Will a portion of the compensation plan include consideration of such non-productivity-based (i.e., value-based) criteria?	
6. Is compensation comparable under both PSA and employment? Are fair market value/commercially reasonable rates under consideration, regardless of the structure? Has an independent valuation expert provided an opinion?	
7. What assurances does the physician group have that the hospital/health system will allow a level of independence and governance, particularly if the structure is the PMA or traditional PSA model?	
8. What is the term of the agreement? More importantly, what are the rights for early termination (with or without cause)?	
9. How much security, both financial and otherwise, will the hospital/health system provide to the practice? What guarantees of income may exist?	
10. What leadership duties and responsibilities will be assigned to the physicians? These may include medical directorships as well as nonclinical leadership positions.	

(Continued on next page)

FIGURE 6.3. PSA Questionnaire *(continued)*

Question	Answer
11. What service line responsibilities and assignments, if any, will the physicians have?	
12. Does the PSA include any wraparounds? For example, are there any clinical co-management or service line management responsibilities? What about medical directorships? Are these enveloped within the PSA or subject to a separate agreement?	
13. Have the strategic, relational, economic, and functional advantages or disadvantages been articulated between the hospital/health system and the practice? Does the employment lite structure allow for full alignment as well as a high level of partnership?	
14. What is the status of the staff and their security, as well as compensation, assuming the traditional PSA is the model of choice? Will there be a guarantee of employment for a post-transaction period?	
15. What are the restrictive covenant/non-compete terms and conditions? Are they different than what an employment model entails?	
16. What are the terms of the employment lite agreement in the context of a changing reimbursement paradigm? For example, if a shift from productivity- to value-based reimbursement occurs, will the increase trigger an automatic change in the compensation structure from productivity to value?	
17. Under the global payment PSA, how is the overhead reimbursed? Is the amount a budgeted total? Is it a fixed amount that is adjusted only upon mutual agreement through a governance committee? Or, is it a combination of a fixed budgeted total to be reimbursed and certain variable expenses tied to wRVUs?	
18. Is the employment lite model a precursor to employment? Is this matter specified in the definitive agreements?	

system or private practice group. These questions and subsequent answers address many, if not all, of the key terms and conditions of a PSA arrangement. The information gathered will facilitate summarizing and analyzing the hospital or practice position before consummating a PSA contract.

SUMMARY

The shifts in the healthcare industry have created widespread changes throughout all components of the business. As a result, many practices and healthcare organizations are seeking ways to improve alignments with other organizations.

PSAs offer a unique way to achieve these outcomes while still capitalizing on the benefits of maintaining a private practice structure. Though they resemble employment at the core, they can serve as a vehicle for alignment among practices and hospitals that are wary of immediately diving into employment. We anticipate PSA arrangements will continue to increase in popularity and stay at the forefront of partnership discussions as healthcare continues to swing toward value.

CHAPTER 7

Joint Equity Ventures

Physicians are paying attention to joint equity opportunities for both ancillary services and practice initiatives. This chapter focuses on noteworthy legal requirements for equity-type structures and addresses opportunities where physicians, hospitals, and private investors may partner.

MODERATE INTEGRATION

As noted in Figure 1.1 (page 2), joint ventures are a moderate form of integration between physician-to-physician organizations, physician-to-hospital organizations, and, increasingly, physician-to-private investor organizations. They are a moderate form of integration because they involve specific initiatives to complete an undertaking that are likely for defined duration periods, and not necessarily permanent. Further, the specific initiative that unites parties under a common enterprise is just that: specific. Alignment is focused on the joint vision and goals of the initiative that brought the two parties together. Byproducts of the initiative may result in additional synergies that promote further alignment between the parties, but that is an indirect benefit of the joint venture that does not carry specific accountability or management focus of the unintended gain, and, thus, is not sustainable under changing circumstances.

Joint equity ventures are a proven affiliation model that physicians have used for years. The promotion of value-based care initiatives opens new opportunities for physicians to affiliate with other physician practices as well as to expand opportunities to affiliate with hospitals/health systems as changing reimbursement and legal constraints promote collaborative care coordination.

Private investors such as private equity firms recognize this changing environment and are expanding affiliation options for physicians as they enter this market. The short- to mid-term nature of joint equity ventures makes it an attractive opportunity for private investors, since they are likely to enter into an agreement with an exit strategy already in mind.

JOINT VENTURE OVERVIEW

In a healthcare context, a joint venture is the pooling of resources among physicians, typically from various practices, with a common interest in accomplishing a desired purpose. For example, this could include real estate initiatives where several physicians pool resources to develop a medical office building in which to house their practices or a sizable ancillary service such as an ambulatory surgery center.

In most instances, a joint venture is considered when the necessary capital is too much for one practice to take on or, in the case of purchasing medical equipment, a single practice does not have the volume needed to operate the equipment at capacity. For example, a gastroenterologist who regularly performs endoscopies could make a substantial profit if he were able to not only receive the professional component reimbursement for performing these services, but also the technical component reimbursement. Although his volume may not justify putting up the capital to build an endoscopy center, he may be able to partner with other gastroenterologists in the area who collectively have enough volume for an endoscopy center to operate at capacity. Alternatively, the physician could look to other specialties in the area and possibly develop a full ambulatory service center.

Some of the key opportunities that typically require a joint venture include:

- Ambulatory surgery center
- Catheterization laboratory
- Dialysis center
- Endoscopy center
- Imaging center
- Infusion center
- Pain management center
- Radiation center
- Sleep study center

This list represents just a few of the possibilities. When it comes to providing designated health services, physicians' involvement in these initiatives is highly regulated by Stark Law and the federal Anti-Kickback Statute. Accordingly, it is essential to ensure legal compliance when developing ancillary services within a practice or through a joint venture.

LEGAL REQUIREMENTS

Physicians and hospitals increasingly are looking for alternative revenue sources to sustain their income. Many of the business models for alternative revenue sources involve joint ventures in the areas of real estate, pharmaceuticals, medical devices, ambulatory surgery centers, durable medical equipment, physical/occupational therapy, imaging, catheterization labs, dialysis centers, endoscopy, infusion, pain management, radiation, sleep studies, specialty hospitals, and more. Before proceeding with any of these ventures, participants would be well-advised to exercise serious due diligence.

From a legal standpoint, the parties must give due consideration to the appropriate state and federal laws and regulations, including the Anti-Kickback Statute, Stark Law, and an array of state-specific laws, among others.

Anti-Kickback Statute Limitations on Joint Ventures

The Office of Inspector General (OIG) has defined a joint venture as "any common enterprise with a mutual economic benefit."[1] A joint venture takes a variety of forms including a contractual arrangement between two or more parties to cooperate in providing services, or it may involve the creation of a new legal entity by the parties, such as a limited partnership or closely held corporation, to provide such services.[2] These joint ventures may be between physicians; physicians and third parties, such as the often-advertised turnkey solutions to certain ancillary services; and physicians and hospitals.

In general, because the OIG views joint ventures with heightened scrutiny, the parties must be careful to consider their liabilities under this statute and whether they can structure the arrangement to afford themselves the protections of an available safe harbor. Safe harbors that are potentially applicable to many joint ventures include the safe harbors for small entity investments, space and equipment rentals, and personal services and management contracts.

The requirements of the Anti-Kickback Statute carve out a safe harbor for investment interests in a small entity.[3] The two most critical and difficult to meet requirements are:

- No more than 40% of the value of the investment interests can be held in the prior year by investors who are in a position to make or influence referrals, furnish items or services to, or otherwise generate business for the entity.
- No more than 40% of the entity's gross revenue related to the furnishing of healthcare items and services in the previous 12 months or fiscal year can come from referrals or business otherwise generated from investors.

The 60/40 requirements listed previously often pose problems for parties trying to protect joint venture arrangements. Therefore, if an ownership interest is involved in the enterprise, the parties will need to consider whether they are able to avail themselves of these protections.

For space and equipment rentals that may be part of a proposed business venture, the rental aspect of the venture must meet the following requirements to fall within the safe harbors for space and equipment rentals:[4]

- The lease agreement is in writing and signed by the parties;
- The lease agreement specifies premises/equipment covered by the lease and precise intervals and charge; and
- The aggregate rental charge is specified in advance consistent with fair market value and does not consider the volume or value of any referrals or business otherwise generated between the parties for which payment can be made by Medicare or a state healthcare program.

Personal services and management contracts are often combined with space or equipment rentals in joint venture arrangements. To obtain the protections of this safe harbor, participants must have in place the following:

- A written agreement is signed by the parties specifying all the services to be provided;
- The term of the agreement is for not less than a year;

- The aggregate compensation set in advance, consistent with fair market value, does not consider the volume or value of any referrals or business for which payment may be made in whole or in part under Medicare or a state healthcare program;
- The services performed under the agreement do not involve the counseling or promotion of a business arrangement or other activity that violates any state or federal law; and
- The aggregate services contracted for do not exceed those that are reasonably necessary to accomplish the commercially reasonable business purpose of the service.

Due to the healthcare industry's shift to less costly care settings, ambulatory surgical centers (ASCs) have continued to rise in prominence and are the basis for many joint equity ventures. The Anti-Kickback Statute provides safe harbor provisions for four categories of ASCs, including surgeon-owned ASCs, single-specialty ASCs, multi-specialty ASCs, and physician/hospital-owned ASCs. For each of the purely physician-owned ASC safe harbors, at least one-third of the physician investor's income from all sources must be derived from the performance of procedures at the ASC. For multi-specialty ASCs, at least one-third of procedures performed by investor physicians must be performed at the investment entity. The OIG has issued several Advisory Opinions regarding ASC ventures, and it is advisable to follow them when pursuing this type of joint equity venture.

Stark Law Limitations on Joint Ventures

Like the Anti-Kickback Statute, Stark Law recognizes certain exceptions such as those for physician services, in-office ancillary services, personal services arrangements, space and equipment rentals, and rural providers.

The physician services exception, along with the in-office ancillary services exception, applies to the referral prohibition for both ownership/investment interests and compensation arrangements. Unlike the Anti-Kickback Statute, Stark Law does not provide an exception for small entity investment interests. This limitation leaves the physician services, in-office ancillary services, and rural provider exceptions as the only likely exceptions for the ownership interest aspect of any joint venture that has an ownership component.

If physician services are furnished by either a member or a physician in the same group practice as the referring physician, under the supervision of a physician who is either a member or physician in the same group practice as the referring physician, they are not subject to Stark's prohibition on referrals. (Note: Physician services is defined here as physicians' services covered under Medicare Part B, whether rendered by the physician or as incident to services that are covered by Medicare Part B.)

The in-office ancillary services exception is relied on heavily by those considering ancillary business ventures. This exception has some specific requirements:

1. The services have to be furnished personally by (a) the referring physician, (b) a physician who is a member of the referring physician's group practice, or (c) an individual who is supervised by the referring physician or a physician in the group practice as long as the supervision requirements are met.
2. The services must be furnished in the same building or a centralized building used by the practice for the provision of some or all the practice's designated health services.
3. The services must be billed by the physician performing or supervising the service, the group practice of which the performing or supervising physician is a member, the group practice of which the supervising physician is a physician in the group practice, an entity that is wholly owned by the billing or supervising physician, or an independent third-party billing company under a contract that meets the personal services exception.

Limitations of Applicable State Laws on Joint Ventures

While the Anti-Kickback Statute and Stark Law are governed by federal law, each state has specific laws that merit special attention by those considering physician affiliation options. To the extent that a joint venture may involve nonphysicians, whether in a management services capacity or as a joint owner, the parties need to consider their state's doctrines against the corporate practice of medicine.[5] In some jurisdictions, the corporate practice of medicine—essentially a prohibition against ownership by a non-physician in an entity that provides medical services—may be in place by statute or common law. Many of these statutes have exceptions that would allow hospitals to employ physicians and/or physicians to provide medical services through a professional corporation or service corporation. In those states that have a prohibition against the corporate practice of medicine, the ban may not be actively enforced. However, in addition to any penalties prescribed by statute or remedies available at common law, depending on the state's medical licensure statutes, the medical licensing board may have the authority to take disciplinary action against a physician's license for violating the prohibition. Therefore, the risk is potentially significant and should be considered carefully.

Physicians and hospitals considering a joint venture must carefully consider the Certificate of Need (CON) laws of their state, if such laws exist.[6] In many states, entities and sometimes physicians are required to obtain a CON to establish certain healthcare services, purchase certain medical equipment, and/or construct or expand a healthcare facility. States have implemented CON statutes to regulate major capital expenditures that may adversely impact the cost of healthcare services, to prevent the unnecessary expansion of healthcare facilities, and to encourage the appropriate allocation of resources for healthcare purposes. As a general matter, these state laws can impose the obligation to obtain a CON prior to operation of the venture. In many states, the process of obtaining a CON can be highly political, costly, and lengthy. In addition to the acquisition of new pieces of equipment or services, some states may not permit joint ownership or leases of the equipment or services with more than one party involved. In other jurisdictions, these types of arrangements may be permitted but may require notification to the appropriate state agency. Compliance with these laws should be added to the physician's due diligence checklist.

Depending on the service(s) provided by the joint venture, the parties involved should check state laws and regulations to determine whether the operation of the venture would be subject to state licensure laws. Typically, these laws require the enterprise to operate the service and/or equipment per specified inspection by state surveyors before and during operation. Prior to proceeding with the project, speaking to the state surveyors is often helpful to be alerted to additional requirements, details, and nuances that may not appear in the statute or regulations.

EQUITY-TYPE STRUCTURES

Joint equity ventures can be structured in several ways. Below are detailed approaches for two of the most common structure models: equity model group assimilation and physician equity.

Equity Model Group Assimilation Approach

An equity model is essentially a more advanced version of a merger, resulting in a jointly owned physician practice. In the true equity model, all of the practice's assets and work initiatives are merged into an equally owned entity between the physicians and the hospital. Therefore, it represents a true partnership between the players.

Unlike a merger in which the hospital invests little capital and has only a minor interest in the entity, a hospital is required to invest a significant amount of capital to fund an equity model. The same applies to the physician group as a virtually equal owner. Also, the equity model often includes the actual professional component of the practice and is not limited to a joint ancillary investment as with a group practice formation.

One of the positive aspects of an equity model is that all the entities—physicians and hospital—are tied by a legal agreement. Because it is a jointly owned single-provider entity, it can easily negotiate contracts with payers. Moreover, it can jointly develop ancillary services, marketing efforts, and an employee benefits package. Having one provider number makes billing easier to administer. Another advantage is the sharing of resources, management, and existing staff within the practice or physician groups.

Because physicians' incomes are based strictly on the performance of the jointly owned entity, all investors share an interest in profitability and return on investment. Typically, the physicians' compensation is based on a professional services agreement or an employment agreement for the services they render. Any operating profit within the entity is distributed in the ratios of equity ownership; however, in some cases, the entity may guarantee the physician employees a certain amount of compensation until the assimilation process is complete, at which point the jointly owned practice must be self-sustained.

Initial investment capital always is a significant consideration in an equity model. Often the practice will be valued, and its value will be a part of the capital that is contributed to the newly owned and established entity.

The challenges of creating an equity model include issues of governance, voting, and control. Additionally, physicians may be daunted by the lack of subsidies or additional support a hospital would offer in a full-employment model. Despite these hurdles, the equity model is one of the stronger joint venture alignment models available to physicians and hospitals.

Physician Equity Approach

Joint ventures often are nonclinical investments such as management services organizations and real estate developments and genuinely add a positive element to the overall physician-hospital relationship. Although the physicians and hospitals are not necessarily adjoined relative to their practices or even the clinical delivery of services, they are truly integrated with such joint initiatives/investments.

Of course, joint ventures often take the flavor of a clinical venture, but they can be difficult from a regulatory and compliance standpoint. Joint ventures as well as other joint ownership arrangements, including the equity models discussed earlier, take on individual deal and loss-specific requirements.

Service provider joint ventures such as ambulatory surgery centers, imaging or diagnostic clinics, and others require equity and capital participation with the opportunity for profit, but also the risk of loss.

The goals of such joint ventures include direct ownership and influence over the service delivery as well as the predictable alignment of interests. Access to capital and return on investment also are goals, especially if the hospital is a deeper-pocketed investor. Often, such joint ventures encompass service line non-compete agreements and can create some other challenges related to the ability to negotiate reimbursement within the joint venture entity and potentially the canalization of market share and return on investment. Nonetheless, the joint venture is often a much better alternative for the involved parties than remaining in competition with one another.

SUMMARY

Though legal requirements can be cumbersome, joint equity ventures are an excellent method of affiliation for physicians to explore with hospitals when employment or other forms of full alignment are not of interest or viable. Traditionally, this has provided a path for physicians and hospital/health systems to collaborate on joint interests where the physicians receive capital and the hospital/health system receives clinical expertise within a defined initiative. These initiatives can serve a strategic need or be circumstantial in nature.

Nonclinical initiatives are prevalent among multiple physician organizations, where joint equity ventures are structured to optimize business opportunities. The industry push to value-based reimbursement creates new business opportunities, and private equity firms spur innovation in this arena where new income opportunities become available, making joint equity ventures an attractive option for physicians to consider for many years ahead.

REFERENCES

1. OIG Special Advisory Opinion. Accessed July 20, 2019. http://OIG.hhs.gov/fraud/docs/alertsandbulletins/042303SABJointVentures.pdf.
2. Federal Register. Special Fraud Alerts. Accessed July 20, 2019. www.oig.hhs.gov/fraud/docs/alertsandbulletins/121994.html.
3. 42 CFR § 1001.952(a)(2)
4. 42 CFR § 1001.952 (b)(c)
5. A listing of corporate practice of medicine states can be found here: Kaiser III, Charles F., and Friedlander, Marvin. Corporate Practice of Medicine. Accessed July 20, 2019. https://www.irs.gov/pub/irs-tege/eotopicf00.pdf.
6. A listing of CON states can be found here: National Conference of State Legislators. Accessed July 20, 2019. http://www.ncsl.org/research/health/con-certificate-of-need-state-laws.aspx.

CHAPTER 8

Private Equity Model for Hospital/Physician Transactions

We discussed in earlier chapters some of the common alignment options available to hospitals and physicians considering affiliations. As we have mentioned, there are many alternatives that both physicians and hospital executives can explore, all of which vary in terms of the degree of affiliation and the terms involved with each of the models. While the employment model has become somewhat the standard for the full integration model, this model continues to evolve and change in terms of structures and approaches.

PRIVATE EQUITY INVESTORS AND THEIR IMPACT ON HEALTHCARE MARKET DYNAMICS

Private equity investors are nothing new to the healthcare world. In the current marketplace, however, we continue to see these actors stimulate change and evolution of the standard transaction structures and approaches to value creation. This activity, in turn, results in more change that trickles down to other players in local healthcare markets and the industry as a whole.

Before we go deeper into the private equity approach and how these actors are spurring change in the current marketplace, let us first define who and what we are talking about when referring to these players. Private equity (PE) firms are investment fund providers that manage large amounts of capital (usually $100 million+ to $100 billion+). The capital is procured from other institutional investors, such as global banks, hedge funds, high net worth individuals, and family offices. Some PE firms are diversified across multiple industry sectors, regions, and the like, while others have a more specialized focus, such as energy, natural resources, real estate, or healthcare.

The investment model behind most PE firms is to deploy capital into a targeted space by acquiring a *platform* company, which is typically the firm's entrance into a specific type of business, market segment, or region. Once this platform is stabilized and optimized to its fullest potential, it will function as sort of a flagship with the primary focus being the launch pad for growth, which will come through add-on acquisitions made by the company. When an appropriate level of growth has been achieved, the PE firm likely will pursue liquidity by selling the company to a larger buyer or through an initial public offering or another transaction.

There are two main points to this discussion. First, we often refer to private equity transactions within the healthcare services space; however, many of these deals occur at the platform level. Why is this relevant? That brings up the second key point, which is that we typically find that the platform acquisition deal entails higher valuations and perhaps more flexible terms, compared to what generally are more standardized and rigid models pursued in add-on acquisitions. This point is critical because in many cases, once the PE firm completes a platform acquisition and implements its operators to stabilize the business and begin pursuing add-on deals, the majority of PE deals are being executed by operating companies that at that point are owned by private equity investors.

Since PE investments are not new to the healthcare industry, why all this discussion about private equity investors relevant to healthcare services entities? It is important to understand that healthcare is fundamentally a local business. Regardless of its structure, ownership, tax status, and players involved, the dynamic between healthcare providers—physicians and hospitals—is centered on local market dynamics.

Based on the current nature of healthcare services, the delivery of medical care not only begins and ends with, but also revolves around clinicians and the organizations under which they operate, including medical practices, hospitals, and other similar entities. Considering this dynamic in terms of the standard hospital and physician practice, it is relatively straightforward, albeit not always without some degree of complexity. However, when the dynamic of an outside party is added, for instance a private equity firm (or PE-sponsored platform) entering into a market with significant capital reserves and in many cases less regulatory constraints, this could result in substantial disruption to what once functioned as a relatively simple local healthcare market dynamic.

This scenario is what we are currently seeing in many markets with PE firms entering and causing significant disruption. This is not to cast a negative light on PE firms and PE-owned entities, which have the right to implement their model where it makes sense; in many ways, this might result in significant value creation and overall economic growth. So, this in no way is meant to imply that PE investors are some big bad wolf trying to impact local healthcare markets negatively. Indeed, disruption can often result in significant value, as we have seen time and again in other industries.

The primary question we raise is how healthcare provider organizations can deal with this type of disruption. How can they continue to remain flexible and dynamic in creating value for their organizations as they confront this evolving market disruption?

THE PE MODEL AND COMPARISON WITH TRADITIONAL ALIGNMENT MODELS

We typically see a few common structures with transactions involving hospitals and physician groups. While hospitals and physicians can pursue many alignment models, the most common transaction structures between these entities are a practice acquisition coupled with physician employment and professional services agreements (PSAs).

As many groups have considered options with potential buyers other than hospitals, there has been a significant increase recently in the number of deals in which practices sell to PE firms or PE-backed platform companies. These deals, however, typically involve very different structures and terms compared to hospital-physician transactions. Below are some of the overarching common characteristics of these different models:

1. **Hospital acquisition of practice coupled with physician employment agreement.**
   a. Acquisition typically includes only tangible assets and hence, minimal upfront money.

   b. Practice can sell any ancillaries separately at fair market value (FMV).
   c. Compensation plan is based on individual physician production with some quality incentives.
   d. Typically, it makes sense for primary care or practices where the priority is reducing risk and attaining more stability in income over upfront dollars.
2. **Professional Services Agreement (PSA).**
   a. Practice maintains independence but there is no upfront money due to no sale of practice; tangible assets could be sold or more likely leased via the PSA.
   b. Practice can sell any ancillaries separately at FMV.
   c. PSA rate is based on a group rate per wRVU; payments can be distributed by the practice.
   d. Typically makes sense only for surgical specialists or proceduralists where reimbursement has declined significantly, and also where ancillary reimbursement has decreased (such as cardiology).
   e. Surgical practices are more likely to have higher value ancillaries (e.g., ASCs), which would allow for upfront dollars if those ancillaries are acquired.
   f. This essentially is the same as going to a single-payer contract where the PSA rate with the hospital ultimately becomes the sole payer (source of revenue).
   g. While maintaining flexibility of how compensation dollars are distributed by the group, the practice still retains risk and overhead obligations through their maintained independence; other typical employment requirements, such as restrictive covenants, are in force.
3. **Private equity acquisition of practice.**
   a. Upfront value (i.e., intangible value or "enterprise value") in the practice is created through the application of a physician compensation reduction.
   b. The compensation reduction ("haircut") is treated as newly created earnings before interest, taxes, depreciation, and amortization (EBITDA), which can then be applied in a discounted cash flow (DCF) model that ultimately determines enterprise value.

c. The haircut is permanent, so the physicians will make less income going forward; however, they would have received the value of that reduced income in the upfront dollars.
d. Some prospective offset to the haircut may be realized via improved access to services and organic growth.
e. The likelihood of the practice being sold soon or possibly experiencing other consolidation based on the new owner's preferences is high.

In the past, hospitals have been reluctant to pay significant upfront dollars to practices, and for good reason. Medical practices fundamentally have no intangible value, as they in effect distribute all their *profits* in the form of excess compensation to their physicians/partners. Because they distribute their earnings to the physician partners as compensation, the FMV of a medical practice typically is limited to tangible assets. This is a regulatory limitation for hospitals; however, it is not something that PE firms or private, for-profit corporate entities are required to follow. Still, they follow it for return-on-investment (ROI) purposes. (Note: The PE model also facilitates succession planning and, thus, is often more appealing to the older physician, five years or less from retirement.)

Recently, however, the perspective has started to shift ever so slightly. This shift is not on the determination of value for medical practices; rather, some hospitals have begun to explore whether they could pursue the same structure as PE firms in their acquisitions of medical practice entities. That means they will not change their position on paying significant upfront dollars tied to intangible value alone; however, hospitals could explore greater upfront money if those dollars were tied to something more tangible, such as the compensation haircut. This is sensible because until now, hospitals have been forced to stand by and watch as PE firms come into their local markets, write large checks, and then implement significant changes that have broader implications (and in some cases adverse effects) on the local healthcare market.

Also, there is a unique component as to how a valuation can be derived with this model that could increase the appeal for physicians to choose to partner in this structure with the hospital over a PE firm (which we address in the valuation section below).

VALUATION CONSIDERATIONS AND KEY DEAL DRIVERS

Before we discuss the valuation in these transaction structures, we must first understand the key drivers of the deal from the perspective of the practice. In evaluating options from the practice's perspective, the most important initial question the sellers must answer is, "Why are they doing this?" More specifically, "What is their greatest priority to achieve in doing a deal?" The buyers must ask themselves whether the main priority for doing a deal is one of the following:

- Maximize upfront value.
- Accept lower upfront value in exchange for more stable income.
- Maintain income but reduce risk of reductions from CMS and commercial payers.
- Remove risk and difficulties of running an independent practice.
- Maintain independence while still achieving greater income stability.
- Partner with another organization to increase opportunities for income diversity.
- Address the needs of succession with the practice.

If the consensus among the physicians selling their practice is to maximize the valuation paid at the time of the transaction and ultimately forego their independence to an outside organization (hospital or PE firm), then the PE model may be the best option. This favorability will increase if the practice is a primary care or a group with few ancillaries. This model likely is the only real option for maximizing upfront value for that type of entity; however, even with ancillaries involved, if the hospital is willing to purchase them, that will only increase the upfront value. Accordingly, this structure becomes even more appealing for surgical specialties.

So how does the valuation work in the PE model? It is a relatively simple approach, although significant technical analyses, modeling, and assumptions are required to derive an accurate dollar amount. In general, these are the key components of deriving enterprise value in the PE model:

1. Determine the haircut (i.e., compensation reduction) to be applied across all physicians.
2. Develop a pro forma financial model whereby the haircut ultimately is turned into EBITDA with growth over a five-year

projection period. (Note: there are critical and detailed steps that must go into the development of these models; however, for this discussion, we assume the model follows all relevant and appropriate standards.)

3. Calculate a DCF valuation model using the financial tenets from the pro forma. This will derive an enterprise value for the entity following appropriate guidelines and standards.

Below is a generic, high-level description of how this process works. The simple illustration in Figure 8.1 relates how the general numbers might fall. (Note: This is a hypothetical example and presented in general form using round numbers.)

FIGURE 8.1. Hypothetical Example of Acquisition by PE Firm

Acquisition by PE Firm		
Practice Revenue		$50,000,000
Total Physician Compensation (Pre-Haircut)		$25,000,000
Total Number of Physicians		10
Haircut	10%	$2,500,000
Reduced Comp per Physician		$250,000
Multiple on Haircut		9
Transaction Value		$22,500,000
Proceeds of Transaction per Physician		$2,250,000

In the example in Figure 8.1, each physician in the group would receive $2.25 million in upfront value for their practice (assuming the proceeds were distributed evenly), compared to the $250,000 in compensation relinquished each year. This model also assumes the PE firm applied a multiple of 9x to the haircut amount to derive their transaction value; however, few true market multiples can be applied for such deal models. As such, applying a multiple against the haircut to derive the value would entail a varied multiple in each transaction based on the financial resources, risk, and flexibility of the parties involved. This valuation calculation would relate solely to the sale of the practice. If the transaction involved the sale of ancillaries or other related entities, such assets would be valued separately and ultimately entail additional value to the sellers in those deals. Typically, the ancillary services would be a separate legal entity, such as an ASC, or for purposes of the transaction, would in effect be treated as such.

As noted, the standard approach for applying this model with PE firms is for the haircut to be a permanent reduction applied throughout the life of the post-transaction relationship in order to validate the upfront dollars. The PE investor requires this action to allow an adequate return on investment over a relatively short timeframe. Then, there likely could be another transaction or liquidity event soon after that.

PRIVATE EQUITY-LIKE MODEL FOR HOSPITALS

There are potential differences for a hospital pursuing a transaction with a practice under a *PE-like* model. A hospital's ROI can be factored in a variety of ways, and in most cases, it would not consider flipping the practice in five or fewer years as a PE firm often does. Therefore, this creates room for flexibility in the structure and economics of a potential transaction.

To compete with PE firms in such scenarios, hospitals must provide more upfront value than is the case with other models. A hospital cannot write the same size check to purchase a medical practice for as high an upfront value as can a PE firm; however, they potentially could present a more appealing offer by implementing the haircut for a defined, limited period, such as three years. So, instead of the physician sellers receiving all their intangible value upfront in exchange for a permanent compensation reduction, they could pursue the same structure where the upfront value is less than a PE offer (though still a significant amount), and their compensation is restored after a relatively short period.

Using the same generic figures from Figure 8.1, the hospital-driven PE model potentially could be as illustrated in Figure 8.2.

In the example, the value of the practice was derived not from using a multiple applied to the haircut, but instead was applied to a DCF model. This is a separate process and one that requires a discussion of its own to fully explain its mechanics and how a valuation is ultimately derived; however, it is a valuation methodology widely used and accepted, if implemented under the proper guidelines and standards.

FIGURE 8.2. Acquisition by Hospital Using PE Model

Acquisition by Hospital Using PE Model		
Practice Revenue		$50,000,000
Total Physician Revenue		$25,000,000
Total Number of Physicians		10
Haircut	10%	$2,500,000
Reduced Comp per Physician		$250,000
Term of Haircut		3
Total Reduced Comp per Physician		$750,000
Multiple on Haircut		N/A
Transaction Value (under DCF Approach)		$19,125,000
Proceeds of Transaction per Physician		$1,912,500

Nevertheless, the value of the practice paid through the upfront proceeds of the transaction is less than the value paid in the PE acquisition.

The more important distinction is that while the physicians received almost $1.913 million in upfront dollars, this amount was attained in exchange for giving up $750,000 of compensation over three years. After Year 3, though, the compensation is restored with appropriate increases, which means that the physicians would continue to benefit from the transaction going forward, more so than if they would have done the same deal with a PE buyer.

SUMMARY

In evaluating this structure, the consideration is what the physician sellers hope to obtain from a transaction. If they want as much money upfront without concern of the impact on future compensation, then a hospital may not be the best option; however, if they seek a significant portion of the practice's value off the table via an upfront distribution of funds while maintaining the ability for this compensation to be restored in the future, the PE-like model could be attractive for both a hospital and the physician group.

CHAPTER 9

Private Equity-Like Transactions

In Chapter 8, we reviewed private equity models, essentially transactions between investor entities (i.e., private equity consortiums) and physician practices. We considered not only the structure of these deals, but also their composition and key terms and conditions. We now explore how such a deal could be replicated between health systems/hospitals and physician groups. Therefore, we identify this model as *private equity-like.*

OVERVIEW OF THE PRIVATE EQUITY-LIKE MODEL

This hybrid model shares several characteristics with the private equity model, but with some key differences. First, this type of arrangement usually is the focus of a sizable specialty practice, generally a group of at least 20 physician partners. The model imitates that of private equity transactions. For example, many private equity transactions involve significant funds paid at the closing, i.e., upfront money. The private equity-like model also follows this pattern.

Most practices distribute all their excess earnings to the partners via compensation bonuses. Thus, it is challenging to generate true earnings based on a multiple of earnings before interest, taxes, depreciation, and amortization (EBITDA) or excess earnings via a DCF, income-approach valuation methodology.

As with private equity structures, private equity-like model transactions convert some of what would otherwise be partner/physician compensation into a bottom-line profit bucket, thus creating profits for deriving upfront value. Comparable to private equity models, this results in a reduction of physician compensation post-transaction. Therefore, the physician-owners realize legitimate funding at closing. Post-transaction, the physicians must take the cut in pay.

Unlike private equity models where this pay reduction continues without interruption, the private equity-like model generally involves a defined, albeit limited, timeframe—usually three to five years—for the compensation reduction. Thus, the upfront money is distributed along with the compensation reduction, although for a defined number of years. After the completion of the specified period, the compensation is reinstated.

Like private equity models, this structure also focuses on the sale of ancillaries and possibly a management services organization (MSO). These entities might be valued separately, depending on their structure and overall make-up. Corresponding to the private equity model, ancillary services such as investments in or complete ownership of an ambulatory surgery center (ASC), MSO, and others, would be a part of the upfront dollars paid at closing attribution.

As with the private equity model, the primary goal is for the parties to work collaboratively to grow the practice's bottom line and have some offset to the reduced compensation.

Figure 9.1 illustrates the private equity-like model. It basically emulates the standard private entity model, except for the time limitation for the salary reduction. Although that reduction could be permanent, it typically is not, to increase the incentive to maintain a long-term relationship between the health system and the practice.

Post-transaction relationships between the parties are similar to other "full" alignment models, such as employment and professional services agreements (PSAs). To be clear, the private equity-like model involves a purchase (or at least a partial purchase, usually majority interest) of the practice. Post-transaction, it includes employment of all the providers (partners, non-partner physicians, and non-physician providers), and all staff. An exception is that the carve-out MSO could be a jointly owned entity between the practice and the health system. In turn, after the transaction, the health system contracts with that MSO for management services.

The private equity-like model allows for governance and overall collaboration of decision making. Further, it accommodates such structures, particularly if a separate MSO, which is jointly owned and contracted by the health system to manage/operate the practice, exists post-transaction. Governance can be structured in a partnering manner like the other employment structures we discuss in these chapters.

WHY DO A PRIVATE EQUITY-LIKE MODEL?

Often, the interest in the private equity-like model stems from its emulation of a standard private equity model; that is, the need for several of the older physicians to realize their ability to "cash-out" their equity. This structure can be challenging because it does not assume the appearance of traditional employment and it involves the payment of significant upfront funds at closing. This stipulation is a major hurdle for both the practice and the health system in that younger physician partners and non-partner physicians have a minimal interest in and generally are averse to compensation reduction. Therefore, the model's compensation reduction may vary by the individual physician and could consider non-physician partners, assuming they can realize some of the upfront money payment, even though they are technically not partners. If necessary, they could be made partners just prior to the transaction.

Also, consideration of upfront money varying by the individual partner, due to the amount of their agreed-upon salary reduction, can create challenges in that generally, such funds are distributed based upon ownership equity where the partners usually possess equal partnership interests.

VALUATION PROCESSES

Now that we have looked at the essential structural components of the private equity-like model let's explore the valuation considerations, especially those related to the practice and how in this model (like the standard private equity model discussed in Chapter 8) are valued for purposes of the transaction.

The valuation process within a conventional private equity model calls for a relatively simple approach. While a great deal of technical analysis, modeling, and assumptions are required to derive an accurate dollar amount, the process is consistent with any other valuation performed on a market or DCF income approach. In general, these are the key components to derive enterprise value in both private equity and private equity-like models:

1. Determine the amount of compensation reduction to be applied across all physicians.
2. Develop a pro forma financial model in which the compensation reduction, or haircut, is ultimately turned into EBITDA, coupled

with growth over a reasonable projection period—typically five years for discounted cash flow (DCF) calculations.

3. Complete the valuation calculation using a multiple of EBITDA and/or DCF income approach. The pro forma will form the foundation of both methods.

As for the private equity-like model, in dealing with a health system, we noted earlier that the amount of the haircut is usually for a limited defined period, whereas under a standard private equity model structure, the physician compensation reduction is permanent. In both cases, the compensation reduction can be mitigated through legitimate growth and expansion capabilities; however, these expectations must be realistic and within reasonable boundaries. In the final analysis, the compensation reduction creates the excess earnings and/or EBITDA, depending upon which approach is used.

A health system pursuing a transaction with a practice under a private equity-like model can encounter several differences. For example, a health system's ROI can be factored in a variety of ways. In most cases, the health system would not consider flipping the practice in five or fewer years, as is typical of a private equity firm transaction; therefore, the outlook is different, which allows room for flexibility in the structure and economics of a potential deal.

Nonetheless, hospitals and health systems in these scenarios must provide more upfront value than under other models to compete with private equity transactions. A hospital cannot merely write the same size check as a private equity (PE) firm to purchase a medical practice for its higher, upfront value. They potentially could present a more appealing offer by implementing the haircut for a defined, limited period, such as three years. So, instead of the physician sellers receiving all their intangible value upfront in exchange for a permanent compensation reduction, they could pursue the same structure where the upfront value is less than a PE offer (though still significant) and restore their compensation after a relatively short period.

The hospital-driven PE model potentially could look like the model illustrated in Figure 9.1.

The valuation illustration in Figure 9.1 would relate solely to the sale of the practice. In an overall transaction, the valuation often involves the sale of ancillaries and related entities such as MSOs. Those entities

FIGURE 9.1. Private Equity "Like" Model

Note—some variables may exist to these components

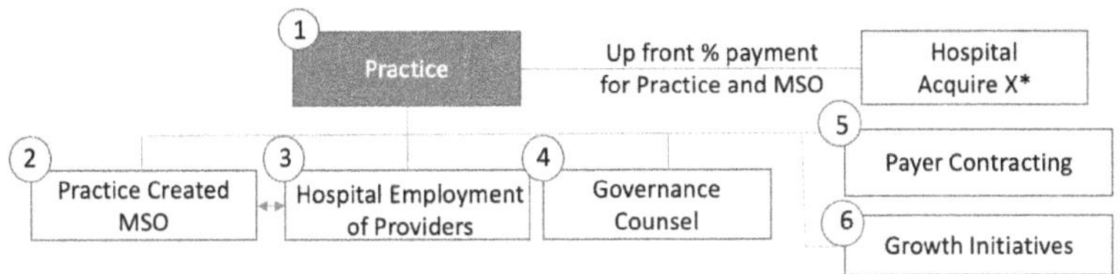

1. Hospital acquires all of Practice via enterprise valuation and none/part of MSO.
2. Practice creates MSO to handle billing and management services and include portion in Transaction (or may exclude and retain all of it).
3. PE-like investment by Hospital in MSO and Practice entails employment of Providers; up-front payment of Valuation Enterprise is created via Providers' post-Transaction compensation reduction; typically the compensation "haircut" is for three years. Pre-Transaction compensation is reinstated after three years. Bottom-line: growth via cost efficiency, revenue enhancement, etc. mitigates the three-year compensation reduction.
4. Practice has representatives on Governance Counsel responsible for communication and organizational initiatives, plus governance/leadership involvement.
5. Practice has access to Hospital payer and other services contracts (via employment).
6. Practice has access to second generation funding for growth initiatives, including ancillary partnership such as ASC investment(s).

** Upfront purchase may be of all/part of the MSO plus **all** of the Practice*

Note: *This model requires careful legal/tax/consulting review as the legal structure of the Practice (i.e., S or C corporation versus LLC) and the treatment of the sales proceeds' being eligible for capital gains tax rates may be in question.*

would be valued separately and ultimately entail additional value to the sellers. Typically, the ancillary services would be a separate legal entity, for instance, an investment in an ASC or, in effect, treated that way for purposes of the transaction.

Figure 9.1 shows that the value of the practice was derived not by using a multiple applied to the haircut, but by using a DCF model, as is generally preferred. This exercise is a separate process that requires a discussion of its own to fully explain its mechanics and how a valuation is ultimately derived; however, this valuation methodology is widely used and accepted if implemented under the proper guidelines and standards.

An independent valuation appraisal expert must be used to perform this analysis and determine a fair market value based on the assumptions of the expected performance and the physician compensation reduction, as well. In this model, the compensation is restored with appropriate increases after Year 3, which also should be reflected in the terms and conditions of the transaction. That is, if the final agreement is for a two-year haircut, then the DCF would be revised to reflect that term.

The private equity-like model has many similarities relative to the derivation of upfront value and payment to the practice. There also are some distinctive differences, not the least of which is the physician compensation reduction for a defined and more limited period. Also, the private equity-like model usually requires less upfront money from the valuation standpoint, as the alignment with a health system can differ substantially from a PE firm. The latter often requires the assumption of significant growth and expansion of other practice acquisitions by the PE firm.

Further, while there are some regulatory and compliance considerations with this type of transaction, they are not as prevalent nor as restrictive, particularly related to the assumptions of growth and expansion that the PE firm often includes within its modeling and valuation calculations.

For example, some PE firms offer additional opportunities to grow and expand, especially if the practice under consideration is "planting the flag" into a particular region, state, or section of the country. Because this opportunity may allow for more growth and expansion, it can be considered in the valuation modeling and upfront value that is derived.

Conversely, health systems have far more restrictions and, from a practical standpoint, would not assume significant growth within its modeling. This is especially true in the typical DCF model where little upfront value typically is derived because all the earnings are distributed and there is relatively minor growth assumed from year-to-year within the projection model (often, 5% or less per year).

Although the similarities between the two models are apparent, the differences in valuation conclusions are significant. These conclusions should be considered in discussing and presenting the private equity-like model to both the health system and the prospective practice.

PROS AND CONS OF THE PRIVATE EQUITY-LIKE MODEL

We have considered the basic tenets of the private equity-like model and have compared it to the standard PE model, noting both similarities and differences. Now, we turn to the principal pros and cons of the private equity-like model.

Pros

1. *Significant upfront payment.* As the model is developed and appropriately structured regarding assumptions of the physician compensation reduction, growth, and other realities of a standard DCF model, it is possible to derive upfront money for the physicians for the practice entity. (Note: If there is a need for capital expenditures, this would be factored into the DCF calculation and thus reduce the value.) This possibility for drawing significant upfront money is unlikely (if possible) in any other model of affiliation and/or full alignment.
2. *Provides a succession plan for the practice.* The provision of succession planning is especially beneficial to older physicians who plan to retire, an eventuality for which many practices are not prepared. This model's allowance for upfront payment provides much more opportunity to accommodate retiring physicians as they transition out of the equity partnership of the practice. Moreover, the structure of the private equity-like model allows for differing amounts of compensation reduction per physician, based on the composition of the bylaws and operating agreement. If the bylaws/operating agreement of the legal entity of the practice will allow, the provision for the upfront money to be paid consistent with the amount of the individual physician compensation reduction further accommodates the succession planning process.
3. *Capital gain income tax rates on the proceeds of the practice sale.* With caution, we emphasize that all transactions should be considered seriously within the context of their overall structure, mechanics, and legal entity formation. There are clear opportunities to treat a portion of the upfront money paid as a capital gain transaction; hence, that gain would be taxed at the lower rates currently allowed by the income tax system. This amount would be in comparison to much higher ordinary income compensation rates.
4. *Long-term employment/alignment.* Like standard employment and even a PSA structure, we consider this a form of "full" alignment, resulting in employment post-transaction. Thus, it allows for the upfront money and the other advantages while still providing the possibility of long-term security and stability.

5. *Opportunity to create other service entities to retain some ownership and infrastructure.* This model allows for the creation or the continuance of an MSO, and potentially other entities that could be jointly owned, such as real estate, medical office buildings, etc.
6. *Joint venture opportunities for ancillaries.* Joint equity venture opportunities are possible, although like every other such transaction, they must be set up with appropriate legal and regulatory boundaries. (See Chapter 7 for further discussion.)
7. *Reinstatement of pre-transaction compensation after the haircut period expires.* In our examples, we have suggested (and therefore used) three years. While this could be for a different period of time, the critical point is that it is a limited/defined period with the possibility for the reinstatement of the pre-transaction compensation foundational totals. This capability is significantly different from a standard PE model where no such assumption exists.
8. *Varied compensation percentage reduction among physician partners.* This model allows for more variety to correspond to the preferences of each physician, giving each the ability to decide how much of a salary reduction they would be willing to assume. It can be drafted to appeal to physicians in all stages of practice in that it allows the flexibility of those approaching retirement to justify a more significant compensation reduction than those who are in earlier stages in their careers and may have more financial responsibilities and commitments.

Cons

1. *Reality of compensation reduction for a defined period.* Though the compensation reduction is for a limited period, it is definitive and must be part of the post-transaction structure. The result is less income to the physicians after the transaction and prior to the restructure.
2. *No assurances during the compensation reduction period that growth will offset compensation reductions.* Similar to a standard PE model, there are no guarantees of growth. While some offsets could occur, generally within a health system transaction, the growth assumptions will be minor, 5% or less per year.

3. *Not as attractive to younger physicians.* Even though the amount of compensation reduction can be less for the younger physicians, the upfront money is less and thus, the overall model potentially not as compelling.
4. *Likelihood of the complete sale of the practice with no retention.* Many physicians would prefer to retain some ownership, which they can generally accomplish with the ancillaries, real estate, MSO, or other components. Nevertheless, it is difficult for them to become full-time employees unless the practice is sold in its entirety. This aspect could be perceived negatively, particularly by younger physicians.
5. *Difficult to unwind once established.* Unwinds are complicated, though not impossible. This dynamic is especially true if the MSO is not created or ongoing as a separate entity, with the physicians having ownership and the ability to take that infrastructure and return it to private practice. Other elements of the unwind can be equally challenging.
6. *Assumption by all physicians of some compensation reduction.* This issue should be evaluated and ultimately decided within negotiations and transaction structuring of the private equity-like model. Generally, however, the expectation is that all physicians will take some salary reduction to be invested in the process. Younger physicians may perceive this negatively.
7. *Possibility that the allocation of the sales proceeds may be in the percentages of the actual equity owned by the partners, not the percentages of the "haircut."* This aspect may mitigate the upfront money receipts and tax effect and should be thoroughly evaluated, discussed, and considered for both compliance and overall structural purposes. There could be issues based upon the legal entity of the practice. For example, S-corporations may require some changes to their inherent structure before completing this transaction. Though other types of entities may be less challenging from a legal structure standpoint, they still present challenges as to how to allocate the sales proceeds and at what tax rate (i.e., capital gains versus ordinary income or a combination of both).
8. *Requirement that there must be "something" for all even though the compensation reduction may vary among physician partners.* Some will consider this issue inherently negative.

9. *Tax and distribution considerations.* Depending upon the structure of the legal entity, there could be greater challenges to framing this model. Even if it is structured legally, some partners who are opposed to the model may oppose proceeding with its application. The practice partners may vote to approve the model, with a majority voting against it.
10. *Capital gains treatment may be challenged.* Capital gains may be deemed appropriate for some or all of the upfront money received, but the Internal Revenue Service could challenge this treatment of the payment as being merely compensation (i.e., ordinary income, taxed) paid upfront as opposed to over a period. Even with the receipt of competent tax advice, this matter has some gray areas.

SUMMARY

The private equity-like model is growing in popularity, primarily because PE firms are becoming more aggressive and doing more deals with physician practices, creating a more competitive environment. It is a viable alternative to hospital/health system alignment transactions with practices, though it is a challenging model to effect. It requires a great deal of planning, discussions, negotiations, and overall structuring that includes significant valuation reviews, post-transaction compensation structuring, and issues related to voting, governance, and distribution of the upfront monies to the partners of the practice. It is not a model for every practice and hospital situation. It is an option to consider and usually applies best to larger single- or multi-specialty practices and health systems that can afford to pay a higher amount of upfront dollars for the practice and invest in other ancillary services. Nonetheless, even though this model presents many challenges, it also offers opportunities to apply the interest that many physicians have in PE models to a similar hospital-alignment strategy. This applies not only to the upfront money but other matters such as governance and income distribution post-transaction, all of which can be favorably structured under this model.

The private equity-like model also requires an ROI for the hospital for those upfront monies. The hospital/health system, therefore, should be able to realize a return on its investment — not just from the "downstream" revenue, but from the transaction itself. Investing in other ancillary entities in addition to the practice acquisition helps in this area. Thus, although the private equity-like model is applicable for some practices and calls for serious study when considering alignment models, it may be quickly eliminated as not viable due to the issues and challenges outlined above. Nevertheless, this model is applicable for some practices and should be considered seriously.

CHAPTER 10

Clinical Co-Management

There are myriad alignment models ranging from full to limited, each offering benefits and challenges. In the moderate category, one of the more prominent models is a clinical co-management agreement (CCMA). CCMAs involve an arrangement between a provider group and healthcare entity (most likely a hospital or health system) for clinical management of a specific specialty or service line. Thus, the providers take an active role in helping the organization meet their clinical goals and advance care for the betterment of the service line.

While this arrangement is common, it often is encapsulated into a broader strategy (i.e., employment, professional services agreement (PSA), and/or clinical integration) and may even be included as a component of that agreement. (Note: Hospitals and health systems are the most common partner for these initiatives; however, they also can be established between provider groups and other institutions, such as skilled nursing facilities and dialysis centers.)

Healthcare continues to move toward value-based care, requiring a dedicated focus of the providers on cost and quality of care. It is imperative, therefore, to have these clinical co-management leaders in place. Now, more than ever, these providers should be considered as part of the overall alignment model. Not only will healthcare organizations and providers benefit culturally and operationally from empowering providers to lead the charge in delivering better quality care, but there can be significant dollars tied to these initiatives (e.g., shared savings) for both parties.

CCMA STRUCTURES

There are four primary categories under which CCMAs fall; however, similar to PSAs, there are infinite ways to develop them to meet the specific nuances of the organizations.

Traditional CCMA

The most common model is the traditional CCMA, where an existing physician professional corporation and a healthcare entity (likely, a hospital or health system) develop a management agreement. This arrangement typically is on behalf of a particular service line, but it also could be for a specific initiative and/or setting of care. The existing professional corporation provides the management services for the hospital's service line. This model is often the easiest to establish as it does not require the creation of a new legal organization. Further, this is most commonly used as an add-on or wraparound for a PSA or other alignment model.

Figure 10.1 illustrates the traditional CCMA structure.

FIGURE 10.1. Traditional CCMA Structure

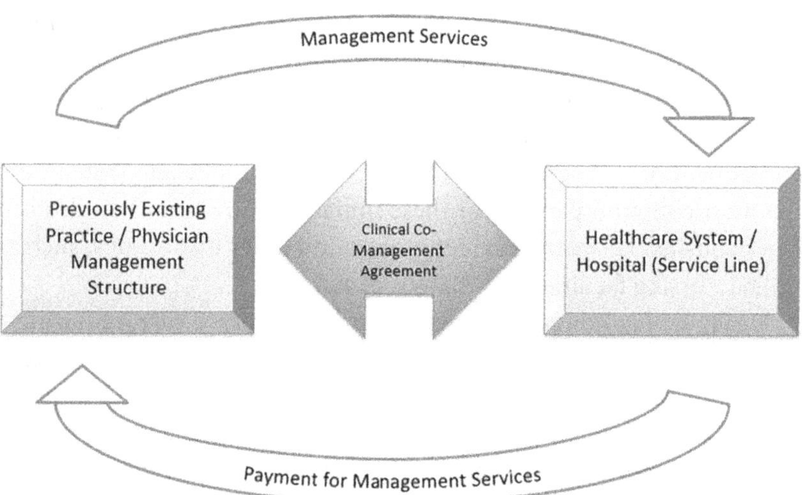

This model most often is established with a single physician group providing the agreed-upon management services to a hospital within a specific service line. The hospital contracts directly with the provider group (as opposed to another entity, as in the other models below). With that said, the hospital may have several CCMAs with provider organizations for different specialties and/or services within the same specialty, although the latter is rare.

This option can be excellent for organizations that want to build a more structured relationship with their provider counterpart without having to align fully and/or change much operationally. If the provider practice has a previously established management entity, this approach is straightforward in developing the management agreement.

If this option is pursued, the organization and the provider group must consider the long-term strategy of the CCMA and establish succession plans for provider-leaders within the CCMA to ensure consistency and longevity of the pursued initiatives.

New CCMA Entity

In this model, a new legal entity is created, which is the entity that contracts directly with the healthcare organization via a management agreement specific to a particular service line(s). In this example, the provider organizations own the new entity, allowing multiple groups to come together under a single umbrella to provide the services. Thus, the healthcare organization would pay the management fee directly to the new entity, which would distribute the funds based on its distribution plan. This model allows for more flexibility in the structure of the CCMA, which opens opportunities for provider groups to join at different times or under different terms, allowing for better succession planning and broader service potentials.

The establishment of the new entity, likely a new PC or LLC, does not need to be overly burdensome or complicated. Usually, this involves working with qualified legal counsel to complete applicable documentation (i.e., state filings, operating agreements, etc.) and paying the associated fees.

This structure works best for healthcare organizations that do not have a single physician entity that is providing the majority of services and/or is seeking to strengthen ties with various provider organizations. In this scenario, the organization would assist in creating this inter-practice dynamic and partnership, although the entity would remain wholly owned by the provider organizations, resulting in stronger ties between those practices as well as to the organization itself.

Figure 10.2 illustrates the newly created CCMA entity.

FIGURE 10.2. New CCMA Entity

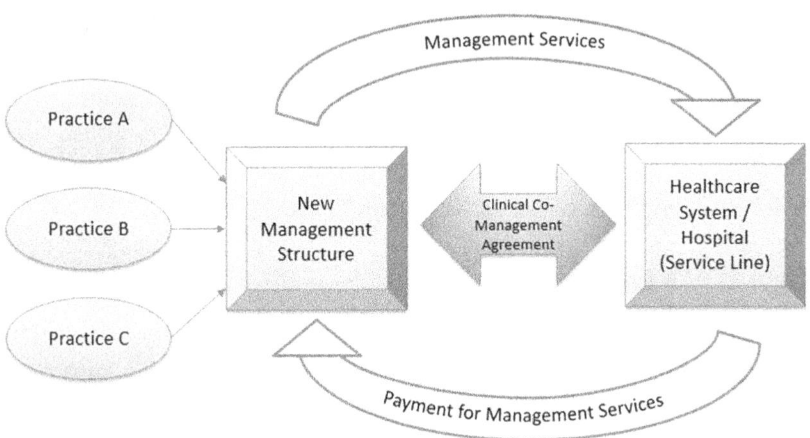

Joint Venture CCMA

This model resembles the new entity model illustrated in Figure 10.2; however, in this scenario, the provider (or set of providers) and a healthcare organization embark on a joint venture to develop the new management entity. This joint venture management entity would then contract directly with the organization for clinical management of a particular service line. Again, the management entity would receive a management fee from the organization and would have authority over distribution among the providers.

The key difference in this example is the level of scrutiny placed on a joint venture and the resulting challenges, including more stringent legal regulations, increased legal fees, extended preparation and implementation time, and more structured requirements for provider organizations seeking to join the joint venture. Thus, this is typically the least-used model for CCMAs and often is only for a specific purpose that cannot be accomplished via the other structures. While it operates much like the new entity CCMA structure, it requires a more permanent alignment between the hospital and physicians, as the management entity is jointly owned (and therefore managed) by the two parties.

Figure 10.3 illustrates the joint venture CCMA structure.

FIGURE 10.3. Joint Venture CCMA Structure

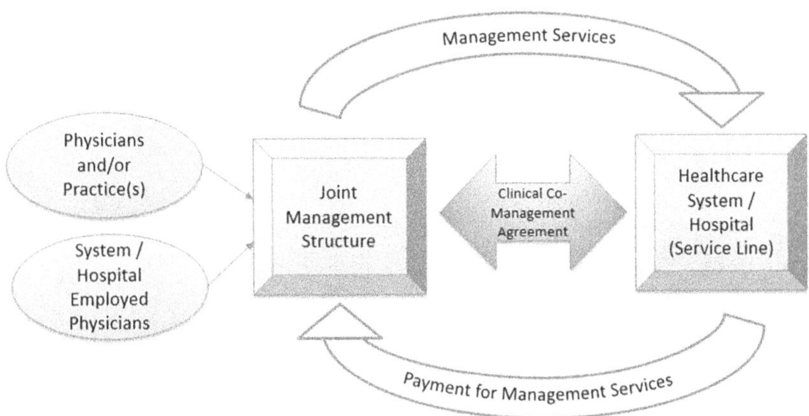

Joint Oversight CCMA

Two or more providers or provider groups, along with their healthcare organization partner, comprise a Joint Oversight Committee in this model. It is important to note that the organization still has single management agreements in place with each group; however, all parties work collectively to meet the clinical, operational, and administrative goals associated with the CCMA for the specific service line.

This model is most like the traditional CCMA in structure (and appears almost identical to outside parties); however, it is developed to support more than one provider or provider group. Another key difference is the role of healthcare organization administrative leadership in addition to the clinical leadership, which may not be required with a traditional CCMA. For providers who wish to use the resources of administrative leaders and/or would benefit from additional oversight, a dyad structure would be particularly fitting.

It is important to note that while the administrative leads would have equal partnership in the CCMA, the clinical leaders would still have oversight and input on key issues. Thus, it may run similarly to a board of managers whereby the different parties generate recommendations on key decisions based on their expertise (i.e., clinical leaders on clinical decisions and administrative leaders on operational decisions). The entire dyad oversight structure casts a vote on the go-forward action plan.

Figure 10.4 illustrates the joint oversight CCMA structure.

FIGURE 10.4. Joint Oversight CCMA Structure

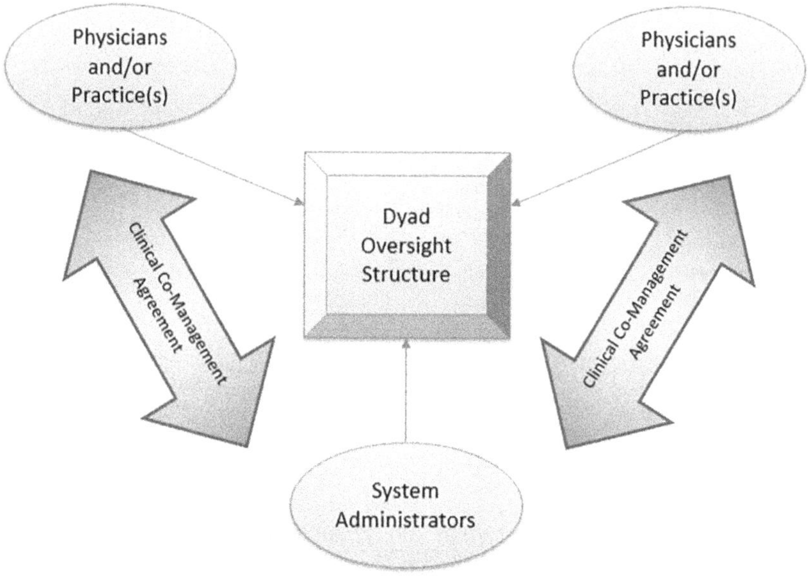

Physicians and/or Practice(s)

Physicians and/or Practice(s)

Clinical Co-Management Agreement

Dyad Oversight Structure

Clinical Co-Management Agreement

System Administrators

CCMA MEASURES

At the core of a CCMA, the healthcare organization typically is typically seeking to achieve certain quality metrics to improve the care for a specific service line. Thus, a comprehensive and collaborative vetting process should be completed before implementation to develop these metrics. This must be a concerted effort between the healthcare organization and the provider-partner to ensure the goals are reasonable and achievable yet challenging enough to drive real change.

Typically, the metrics focus on quality improvement, provider accountability, coordination of care, physician leadership, and value-based goals. Moreover, these should have clear baselines and targets associated with them to ensure the organization can attribute specific successes to the CCMA. These should become more aggressive over time, with the initial years focused on more attainable targets to set the foundation and the future years focused on improving upon previous success. Additionally, the metrics should be established to allow for flexibility as the CCMA grows and matures (i.e., patient volume, provider participation, etc.).

The healthcare organization must use historical performance data to set the baseline for these metrics. Precedent in these arrangements has mandated that any financial incentives tied to these programs consider the healthcare organization's historical data in establishing the specific baselines to ensure that the CCMA is, in fact, the driver of these changes. Additionally, having access to this data before setting the metrics can highlight where to place the focus.

Examples of applicable metrics include:

- Patient access
- Panel size
- Outcomes
- Use of extenders
- Care coordination
- Medical home concepts
- Patient satisfaction
- Cost containment

As with any arrangement, the CCMA should allow the metrics and benchmarks to be updated consistently (typically annually) to correctly align the goals of the healthcare organization, current market trends, and the outcomes of the CCMA.

FEE STRUCTURE

CCMAs typically consist of two separate components of pay for participating providers. The first component is the annual base fee, which is fixed and substantiated by fair market value. Most often, this is based on hourly rates for similar services as opposed to the achievement of specific metrics. Thus, this takes into consideration the time and effort of the provider's services associated with the CCMA, and, specifically, the service line development, management, and oversight.

Additionally, a component of compensation is tied to the achievement of previously agreed-upon quality, cost, or operational metrics. Thus, these are explicitly linked to the metrics highlighted above, basing success on the baselines and targets established in the CCMA. This portion of the CCMA can be very lucrative depending on the metrics and may allow for significant upside for both the hospital and the provider organization, for example in the case of shared savings.

PROS AND CONS

As with all alignment models, there are benefits and potential drawbacks to consider before enactment. Figure 10.5 illustrates a non-exhaustive list of these factors for organizations to study when pursuing a CCMA.

A CCMA is a viable solution to many of the challenges healthcare organizations struggle with relative to value-based care and running a successful service line. It draws upon the clinical expertise of its providers while providing significant financial and operational rewards to those providers for their role in the organization. CCMAs are growing in popularity but remain underutilized, especially as healthcare organizations continue to be pressured for higher quality and lower costs. CCMAs are excellent in driving cooperation and coordination between provider groups and their healthcare partners without requiring significant structural ties. They must be considered carefully, however, as they do require concerted efforts from both administrative and clinical leaders. Regardless, for highly autonomous providers, a CCMA may be a more desirable approach to healthcare partnership as it maintains high levels of independence and empowerment both in their own practice and in the healthcare organization itself. With that said, the CCMA is typically not a long-term partnering solution and will usually end in a shift to a more fully aligned model.

SUMMARY

As the healthcare industry continues to emphasize the importance of valuable care, and as patients become educated consumers, it will be imperative that healthcare organizations understand the importance of provider leadership in driving change to their frontlines and be willing to invest in these efforts.

CCMAs offer a unique approach to alignment, allowing for providers and healthcare organizations to work collaboratively to meet mutually beneficial outcomes. They also can serve as the foundation for more substantial alignment models, demonstrating how the relationship may look under future arrangements.

FIGURE 10.5. Pros and Cons of a CCMA

Benefits	Considerations
• Can be included as an *add-on* or *wraparound* to an existing or new overarching alignment strategy (i.e., employment or PSAs) • Uses clinical leadership to advance key goals/objectives of the organization that relate to the quality, cost, and management of services • Easily customizable to address preferences of all parties involved • Value of CCMA can range from relatively insignificant dollars to material figures • Better prepares all organizations to meet the increasing demands of value-based care • Can offer a *win-win* solution for providers and heatlhcare organizations where providers are given an opportunity to participate in fee-for-value reimbursement models without investing significant amounts of capital, and hospitals are able to utilize provider influence and clinical insight to control costs and improve quality • Allows physician to be in the *driver's seat* and, thus, better engaged in the movement to reduce cost without compromising care quality • Supports a collaborative and highly engaged culture • Allows for scalability and supports the development/success of models such as ACOs, PCMHs, and CINs	• Entails a cultural shift that relies upon transparency, open communication, data utilization, and collaboration • Entails additional investment of resources (financial, time, and energy) to first develop the CCMA and then sustain it over time • Can lead to *physician fatigue* or relational issues if improperly structured • While technically possible, seldom a long-term standalone strategy (i.e., will require a broader alignment/clinical integration plan for the outlying years)

CHAPTER 11

Limited Affiliation Structures

In Chapter 1, we presented an overview of the past 50 years of physician affiliation models. This brief history highlighted several trends in affiliation structures that shifted between limited, moderate, and full integration at various points from the 1970s to the second decade of the 21st century.

Recently, the regulatory environment and value-based payment movement have caused affiliation structures to favor moderate to full integration. Other chapters describe these moderate to fully integrated affiliation models; this chapter will focus on some of the limited affiliation options available to physicians and health systems.

As mentioned in Chapter 4, Limited Integration models entail relationships among the relevant parties that stop short of significant long-term integration/affiliation and involve minimal negotiation. The options we will discuss in this chapter include either task-oriented relationships or memberships with loose alliances among physicians and/or hospitals. Included is an outline of the basic structure and intent for each alignment example within the Limited Integration portion of Figure 11.1, except Group Mergers, which will be described in further detail in Chapter 13.

After a description of each limited affiliation model, the chapter concludes with a review of compliance considerations important for physicians and health systems to discuss as they consider or negotiate such options.

MEDICAL DIRECTORSHIPS

Medical directorships are a long-standing but limited form of integration between physicians and health systems. In these affiliation models, the physician is contracted through a professional services agreement

FIGURE 11.1. Traditional Alignment Model Descriptions

Limited Integration	Moderate Integration	Full Integration
Managed Care Networks (Independent Practice Associations, Physician Hospital Organizations): Loose alliances for contracting purposes	**Service Line Management:** Management of all specialty services within the hospital	**ACO/CIN/QC:** Participation in an organization focused on improving quality/cost of care for governmental or non-governmental payers; may be driven by practices or hospital/groups
Recruitment/EPPM/PSM: Economic assistance for new physicians	**MSO/ISO:** Ties hospitals to physician's business	**Employment "Lite":** Professional services agreements (PSAs) and other similar models (such as the practice management arrangement) through which hospital engages physicians as contractors
Group (Legal-Only) Merger: Unites parties under common legal entity without an operational merger	**Clinical Co-Management:** Physicians become actively engaged in clinical operations and oversight of applicable service line at the hospital	**Employment*:** Strongest alignment; minimizes economic risk for physicians; includes a "PE-Like" model
Call Coverage Stipends: Pay for unassigned ED call	**Joint Ventures:** Unites parties under common enterprise; difficult to structure; legal hurdles	**Group (Legal and Operational) Merger:** Unites parties under common legal entity with full integration of operations
Medical Directorships: Specific clinical oversight duties		**Private Equity Affiliation:** Ties entities via legal agreement; sale to private investor/operator

Legend: Typically Physician-to-Physician; Typically Physician-to-Hospital; Either Physician-Physician or Physician-Hospital; Physician to Private Investor

* *Includes the Physician Enterprise Model (PEM) and the Group Practice Subsidiary (GPS) model both of which allow the practice entity to remain intact even after employment of the physicians by the hospital*

(PSA) to provide clinical oversight for a particular department, service line, or other operation within the system. Each arrangement typically involves compensation paid at a specified hourly rate with monthly or annual limits on the number of hours committed or total compensation paid.

Additionally, the health system creates a job description for the medical director position that outlines the relevant responsibilities, tasks, projects, service line or department performance measures, etc., for that role. Many of these arrangements have short terms (one to three years) that will renew automatically or be renegotiated after the initial term, as is the case with more robust PSAs.

While some physicians are not interested in moderate or full integration with health systems, medical directorships might be an attractive alternative for them because they provide additional compensation at fair market value (FMV) and foster stronger engagement with health system initiatives. On the other side of the table, medical directorships allow the health system to maintain or more effectively manage a needed service for a reasonable price and limited downside risk.

Health systems, given their limited scope, should not consider medical directorships alone as an alignment model that will promote or develop broader integration structures (i.e., ACOs or CINs); however, physicians find that such relationships are still relevant and vital as they become more engaged in administrative capacities to effectuate necessary changes in a more value-based healthcare environment.

CALL COVERAGE ARRANGEMENTS

Pay-for-call is a popular form of compensation for physicians who serve in the hospital's emergency department (ED) call rotation and are directed to unassigned patients who present in the ED. Unfortunately, as payer mix challenges have increased, the number of paying patients in the ED has diminished dramatically. The average ED patient is often uninsured, self-paying, or non-paying. Therefore, physicians covering call without pay sacrifice their time and income on many levels.

Under the federal Emergency Medical Treatment and Labor Act (EMTALA), hospitals are bound to provide care for all individuals who appear in their ED. Physicians not bound by EMTALA, however, are less willing to provide patient care without some compensation. For these reasons, more physicians are receiving remuneration from hospitals for being on call.

Physician on-call compensation varies widely, but a few of the primary mechanisms include hourly rates, daily stipends, monthly or annual stipends, and per-procedure/case compensation. Most arrangements involve either hourly rates or daily stipends. According to the Medical Group Management Association's (MGMA) 2018 Provider Compensation and Production Survey, approximately 31% of their survey respondents reported hourly rate on-call compensation and 38% reported daily stipend compensation.[7]

Similar to medical directorships, on-call agreements are generally one to three years in duration and may renew automatically after that. The level of compensation paid is driven primarily by the burden that the call responsibilities place on the physician. This burden can be determined by the length of the call shift, whether the provider is required to be at the hospital during their shift, how many call occurrences take place, the acuity or level of complexity of the patients served, the proportion of uninsured or underinsured patients, and the response-time requirements for the physician. In general, higher call burden and more complex environments of care, like trauma centers, will create the need for higher call compensation rates for physicians.

On-call agreements offer physicians an option for additional compensation beyond their practice operations and provide a narrow scope of responsibility and limited opportunity for alignment with a health system; however, this particular alignment alternative might serve as a productive first step for physicians or health systems seeking broader integration in the future.

RECRUITMENT ASSISTANCE

Another limited alignment option involves a hospital providing financial assistance as an incentive in recruiting physicians to join one of the private practices in its geographic service area. While this type of arrangement can pose a potential risk for Stark Law violation, there is an exception that addresses physician recruitment explicitly. This exception allows for such relationships between hospitals and private practices when hospitals can justify both a community need and benefit from the recruited physician's specialty. It is important to note that the exception applies only to hospitals, federally qualified health centers, rural health clinics, and providers joining an established medical group.[8]

Although this process is subject to substantial regulatory scrutiny, it has traditionally been a major form of alignment, although limited, between hospitals and private practices. Because the recruited physician enters private practice, he or she is not directly integrated (at least long-term) with the hospital or health system. Moreover, that physician is not obligated to work with that hospital. Further, the recruitment guarantee loan is forgiven entirely as long as the physician continues to work in the service area, not in any particular hospital.

Another option for recruitment assistance is the incubation model in which the hospital employs the physician for a limited period—usually one to three years—and then places him or her in the private practice without full alignment or integration with the hospital. Despite the limited nature of this alignment option, recruitment assistance can provide physicians in private practice significant value with minimal risk.

These arrangements allow private practices to continue to function independently while providing the hospital an opportunity to serve patients more adequately within its geographic region. Successful recruitment assistance relationships can help build trust and ultimately lead to more moderate or even full integration models in the future.

MANAGED-CARE NETWORKS

Managed-care networks are a basic form of limited alignment, usually established through independent practice associations (IPAs) and/or physician-hospital organizations (PHOs). IPAs, as defined by the American Academy of Family Physicians (AAFP), are "business entities organized and owned by a network of independent physician practices for the purpose of reducing overhead or pursuing business ventures such as contracts with employers, accountable care organizations (ACO) and/or managed care organizations (MCOs)."[9] PHOs are very similar to IPAs, but instead of physicians aligning with other independent practices, they align with other physicians and hospitals to form a network that can share information, care coordination capabilities, and leverage size and quality in contracting negotiations. Both IPAs and PHOs can qualify for consideration as ACOs under the Affordable Care Act (ACA) or can serve as critical foundations for broader CINs.

Physicians who consider joining an IPA or PHO should understand membership requirements and costs as well as the overall strength of the organization's leadership. In the past, IPAs and PHOs represented very loose affiliations that may not have effectively integrated the member organizations around the quality of care, population health management, or cost management. Managed-care networks offer independent practices a reasonable option to affiliate with a broader network while maintaining almost all autonomy.

In today's healthcare landscape, it would be prudent for an independent practitioner to consider partnering with such entities even if they prefer to not align more closely with a hospital or health system in their service area.

SUMMARY

As with many of the other affiliation strategies described in this book, it is vital for physicians and hospitals or health systems to carefully consider all legal and compliance implications before pursuing a specific alignment model. Regarding the Limited Integration models reviewed in this chapter, FMV evaluations should be completed by a third party for medical directorships and call coverage arrangements. Also, parties should consider commercial reasonableness as well as any potential financial conflicts of interest or the perception that an agreement is struck with the intent to steer patient referrals or designated health services to a specific entity in the area. Many of these critical questions can be answered with the help of outside legal counsel or healthcare appraisal services.

Once all compliance risks have been considered and addressed, limited forms of alignment can serve as a productive first step toward broader integration for independent physicians and hospitals or health systems. At a minimum, the models reviewed in this chapter provide some targeted win-win scenarios for all parties involved without sacrificing autonomy on the physician side or creating significant financial or compliance risk on the hospital side.

REFERENCES

1. Medical Group Management Association. 2018 Provider Compensation and Production Report: Based on 2017 Survey Data. Group Demographics – On-Call. MGMA.2018.Accessed June 28,2019.https://data.mgma.com/DataDive/Documents/OC%202017%20Demogs.pdf?.
2. Champion S, Kiehl D. Guidelines and Strategies for Navigating Stark's Physician Recruitment Exception. Coker Group Whitepaper. 2016. Accessed June 28, 2019. https://cokergroup.com/wp-content/uploads/2016/11/Physician-Recruitment_November-2016.pdf.
3. American Academy of Family Physicians. Independent Physician Associations (IPAs) Defined. AAFP website. Accessed June 28, 2019. https://www.aafp.org/about/policies/all/independent-physicianassoc.html.

CHAPTER 12

Clinically Integrated Networks and Value-based Reimbursement Affiliation Models

Historically, doctors have affiliated with hospitals and with other practices, but the reasons for the affiliations have changed significantly during the past decade. Hospitals and physicians traditionally have partnered for practical purposes—the hospital served as the physician's workshop for patients requiring inpatient care.[1] The hospital's medical staff worked to ensure that only qualified, appropriately credentialed physicians were given privileges to practice in the facility. Rarely, in this model, did the hospital and medical staff align for the purposes of improving quality or patient safety, and even more rarely did the hospital actually employ physicians with the exception of hospital-based specialists such as pathologists or radiologists. In addition, physicians who were not part of the same professional group or firm seldom banded together in meaningful ways. Legal and regulatory barriers, particularly those related to anti-trust regulation, made such affiliations especially rare.

Until recently, when the imperative to improve quality and reduce costs became paramount, affiliations between various kinds of healthcare providers were only loosely organized and failed to align or integrate these providers in a significant fashion. Evidence of this can be seen in the failure of most hospital medical staffs to police the practice patterns of physicians given privileges to practice in the hospital.

With the 1999 publication of the Institute of Medicine (IOM) report "To Err is Human," which included the rather shocking statistic that nearly 100,000 Americans die each year due to medical errors, quality improvement efforts began to move forward in most hospitals, but it quickly became evident that these efforts would not succeed without the full engagement of the medical staff.

A little more than 10 years after the publication of the IOM report, the cost of care in American healthcare facilities joined quality improvement as a major focus of attention and resulted in significant reform efforts, particularly at the federal level as reflected in the passage of the Affordable Care Act (ACA) in 2010. Again, most hospitals and even smaller facilities realized that without physician alignment and engagement, cost-control efforts would fail.

Thus began the era of value-based healthcare delivery, where value is defined as *quality measures per unit of cost* and the overarching imperative in the system has become the *simultaneous improvement of quality outcomes and lowering of costs*. One of the pioneers in this area was the Advocate Health System in Chicago, which argued that physicians who are clinically integrated (as defined by the Federal Trade Commission and others) could legally band together for contracting purposes in order to improve value production in healthcare.[2]

Producing higher quality and cost efficiency, however, has not been easy, nor has it been easy to bring the requisite players to the table—especially physician providers—to achieve this essential goal. One of the primary reasons for this failure to move the dial related to quality and cost is the lack of effective venues or affiliation models within which meaningful strides toward higher value can occur. Physician practices, hospital medical staffs, even staff model or clinical model HMOs have not been successful in this regard.

This chapter will examine some of the other structures that have been devised to deliver higher value within the healthcare system. While the verdict is still out as to which of these existing models will succeed and what future models might be required to truly deliver high-value care, all providers of healthcare services must understand how the demand for value is driving change at the organizational level. Before outlining the structures or organizations that are now being used to drive higher value, we will first consider the payment models that are also driving significant change across the healthcare industry.

VALUE-BASED HEALTHCARE REFORMS

Payment for healthcare services traditionally has been on a fee-for-service model wherein specific cognitive or procedural services are paid for directly or indirectly by third-party payers on a piecemeal basis. An example of this is when, after a doctor's office visit, the patient or his or her insurance company is sent an itemized bill for evaluation and management services and any associated procedures (injections, tests, radiographs, minor surgeries, etc.) performed at the time of the visit.

Attempts to change the above model of payment first came about in the 1980s and 1990s with the advent of managed care. Here, primary care gatekeepers were contracted through a capitation model to manage the care of patients for whom they were then held responsible for both clinical and financial outcomes. A capitated payment was rendered prospectively to the provider on a per-member per-month basis (PMPM) and the costs of all qualified services provided to the patient were then deducted from that capitated payment. At the end of the designated period, usually one year, any dollars left over in the payment account accrued to the provider, ostensibly for managing the care of the patient in a cost-efficient manner during that time. Conversely, if the costs of care exceeded the cumulative PMPM payments, then the provider was at risk for paying these excess costs back to the payer.

Capitated managed care has, for the most part, vanished from the U.S. insurance system mostly due to dissatisfaction by providers who felt that they were being forced to assume more risk than they were prepared to manage. Likewise, patients thought that the capitated care arrangements created perverse incentives that rewarded cost control over high-quality care delivery.

More recent alternatives to fee-for-service care delivery include a variety of so-called value-based reimbursement models, all of which attempt to drive higher value care delivery by rewarding not only quality of care but also cost-efficient care. These models differ in many ways, but their standard components include:

1. Quality outcome measurements specific to the services rendered, such as Hemoglobin A1C levels for diabetic patients, with the setting of measurement thresholds that must be met before payments are rendered.

2. Cost-of-care measures which, when compared to historical cost payments, can result in a cost savings bonus that is shared by the payer and the provider. (Note: The patient rarely gets a rebate or discount when savings result.)

An example of such a reimbursement arrangement would be a bundled payment for the care of patients undergoing orthopedic total joint replacement surgery.[3] Here, each of the individual providers along the care continuum, from primary care to surgeon, to hospital, to rehab facility, and others are paid on a traditional fee-for-service basis for the care rendered to the patient. At the end of the measurement period, however, if the payer's costs (the cumulative total of the fee-for-service payments) is less than projected *and* if the providers achieve certain quality measurement thresholds, such as the number of patients with complications or readmissions, then savings are shared between the payer and the providers, usually on a 50/50 basis. The way the providers then allocate their 50% share of the savings depends on pre-determined income distribution plans set by the providers, and this then depends on how, and if, the providers are affiliated with each other.

The quality measurement thresholds that must be achieved prior to the payment of shared savings bonuses are considered a major step toward correcting one of the primary deficiencies of capitated managed-care contracts in the 1980s and 1990s. In these older arrangements, many providers could simply say no when it came to approving emergency room visits, hospitalizations, tests, or procedures. By doing so, they generated savings for themselves and the payers, and patients often suffered the consequences of lacking access to necessary care.

However, the core problem is that the definition of a high-quality outcome and the measurements that reflect this goal differ considerably between payers and providers and among individual providers. Also, the system's ability to measure outcomes, particularly those related to quality, is limited and in its nascent stages. Many providers, therefore, feel that basing reimbursements on quality measures is putting the cart before the horse and they should not be held accountable for achieving that which cannot be measured accurately.

ORGANIZING AROUND VALUE-BASED REIMBURSEMENTS

As the above example shows, contracting for value-based reimbursements (VBRs) can create many opportunities for providers (individuals and institutions) to affiliate in novel ways. Using the example of bundled payments for orthopedic surgeries, the providers and facilities involved may want to unite to have a formal venue through which they can design high-quality, cost-efficient processes of care, measure quality and cost outcomes, market services, and contract with payers or even large self-insured entities.

These affiliations are referred to by several names, including accountable care organizations (ACOs), clinically integrated networks (CINs), physician-hospital organizations (PHOs), independent provider or physician associations (IPAs), and others. While each of these affiliations may differ in some details, their common purpose—to jointly contract on behalf of otherwise non-affiliated providers for value-based reimbursements—is the same.[4]

There has been tremendous growth of these types of organizations during the 10 years since the passage of the ACA, which also included the creation of Medicare ACOs. The most common corporate structure use for this purpose is the single or multi-member limited liability corporation (LLC), which is easy to create. What is not so easy to develop are the governance and operational rules around the organization, especially since most of these entities bring together rather disparate groups of providers all of whom have not previously shared the same tax identification number (TIN).

For example, a bundled payment orthopedic contracting entity might bring private practicing orthopedists, anesthesiologist, and rehabilitation medicine specialists together with for-profit or not-for-profit hospitals and rehab facilities. The good news is that many of the restrictions on joint contracting by these entities have been lifted vis-a-vis anti-trust concerns, but those providers who want to join such affiliations would still be well-advised to seek qualified legal counsel before entering a CIN, IPA, or other such entity.[5]

Some of the more controversial topics that value-based reimbursement affiliations (VBRAs) such as CINs or ACOs need to consider are:

1. **What is the governance structure of the VBRA?**
   Most such entities create a governing board with representation from the principal players in the VBRA (individual physician practices, hospitals, ancillary service providers, etc.). This board not only governs but also manages the VBRA via sub-committees that usually include:
   - Payer Relations Committee—responsible for negotiating, contracting, and managing payer agreements on behalf of the VBRA.
   - IT Committee—responsible for determining the IT infrastructure the VBRA will need and selecting specific vendors to meet those needs.
   - Provider/Professional Assessment Committee—responsible for reviewing data regarding the quality and cost efficiency performance of each provider in the VBRA and setting standards, which must be met to avoid remediation by the VBRA, ultimately to include expulsion of poor-performing providers.
   - Executive Management Committee—responsible for making day-to-day decisions regarding the VBRA. This committee usually includes the board chair, vice-chair, and secretary.

2. **Who will own the VBRA?**
   Most of these organizations are not set up to be profitable enterprises but, instead, are vehicles through which their members can respond to the increasing numbers of value-based reimbursement agreements available in the marketplace. Perhaps more importantly, they have a venue wherein the members can create high-value (quality per unit of cost) integrated care processes that can deliver on these contracts. Therefore, the question of who owns the VBRA becomes less important than how well it functions and can provide high-quality at low cost to the payers and ultimately, the individual patients they serve.

3. **How will the VBRA hold its members accountable?**
   To avoid unwelcome scrutiny from the Federal Trade Commission (FTC) regarding anti-trust issues, a VBRA must have a system whereby it not only tracks quality and efficiency but holds its members accountable for increasing quality and decreasing costs.

   Traditionally, hospital medical staffs and even private group practitioners have not done a good job regarding such *peer review* activities. Therefore, one of the tasks of a well-functioning VBRA will be to put *the accountability into accountable care.* Actions to hold providers accountable for their performance within a CIN should be spelled out beforehand and may include termination from the VBRA for those who fail to perform up to standards consistently. Interestingly, this rarely is necessary. Less egregious methods of holding providers accountable, such as regularly notifying them of how they are performing against their peers or simply using carrots instead of sticks (e.g., higher bonus payments to top performers), results in consistent improvement efforts by most participants.

4. **Will opting out of certain contracts be an option for some providers?**
   VBRAs, especially those that are just starting, may be tempted to allow participating providers to opt out of certain contracts. This should be avoided, as it will diminish the negotiating leverage that these groups have with payers and may lead to disharmony and dissension within the organization. Especially at first, the VBRA should strive for a unified approach to contracting.

5. **How will revenues be shared within the VBRA?**
   When received, revenues such as shared savings bonuses will need to be distributed among the providers within the VBRA. A fair and equitable system for doing this needs to be created up front to avoid discord within the group, especially that which may result if some participants believe that others are not contributing to the success of the group and, instead, getting a free ride by the VBRA.

   The most important point, however, is that the income distribution plan needs to be decided before there is any income to distribute to avoid an even bigger conflict when revenues are earned and there is no pre-determined way to divide them among the providers.

6. **How will the VBRA be financed?**
   Forming even a small VBRA can be quite an expensive proposition. IT infrastructure, management staff, office space, and the time/opportunity costs of those participants who must organize

and manage the VBRA are all expenses that must be considered. For this reason, many organizations of this type are financed by hospitals or healthcare systems, which have more resources and existing infrastructure and staff that can be used for this purpose.

Putting together a hybrid organization where the hospital/healthcare system pays all the bills but the independent providers govern the entity (the FTC states that a CIN must be physician-led) can be difficult to accomplish. Within many communities there is significant distrust between the hospital and its medical staff; therefore, physicians tend to worry that when the hospital foots the bill to create a VBRA, they will want to control its operations. Similarly, the hospital may feel that it is unfair for them to have to put up the money to get the VBRA off the ground and then turn over the governance to the physicians.

There are many instances where this kind of distrust has run nascent CINs and ACOs off the rails. However, there are also examples of hospitals and providers overcoming these obstacles and achieving mutual success through the creation of a highly functioning VBRA. The old saying that a rising tide lifts all boats applies here. Thus, the emphasis should be that in a value-based reimbursement environment, all providers (physicians, hospitals, health systems, and ancillary providers) will benefit by integrating their efforts, both financial and clinical.

7. **Who will be the marketing targets for VBRAs?**

   Many payers, both commercial and governmental, have introduced value-based payment models to include:

   - CMS:
     1. Medicare Accountable Care Organizations (ACOs) operating through the Medicare Shared Savings Programs (MPPS)
     2. Medicare Access and CHIP Reauthorization Act Payment Models
        a. Merit-based Incentive Payment System (MIPS)
        b. Alternative Payment Models (APMs)
     3. Bundled Payment Care Improvement (BPCI) Programs
   - Commercial
     1. ACOs
     2. Bundled Payments

Additionally, VBRAs will need to consider marketing their services directly to large self-insured employers such as Walmart, Lowe's, Home Depot, and others.

Finally, many single specialty VBRAs (orthopedic, ophthalmology, etc.) may find that they can contract with other VBRAs through so-called wraparound agreements where they fill in the specialty gaps that may exist in one or more local ACOs or CINs.

CARE PROCESS DESIGN

The other major task confronting every VBRA is how to redesign frontline care delivery so that it reliably produces higher quality at lower costs. This task is not easy either, especially given that the practice patterns of most healthcare providers have been left up to their own discretion and not rigidly controlled by outside interests. The central feature of value-based reimbursements, however, is that they can entice providers to change their actions by offering payments for objectively measured outcomes (quality and cost) rather than objectively defined services.

The problem is that for much of what is done in healthcare delivery, there is no hard evidence that one method of delivering care is better than another. Instead, many practice patterns are based on habits, customs, and what seems intuitive to individual practitioners. While most physician providers claim they worship at the altar of evidence-based medicine, the truth of the matter is that there is very little evidence for most of what is done in healthcare. This will have to change and hopefully some of the outcome measurements usually reserved for clinical/scientific studies will now be generated in the payer realm and drive improvements in day-to-day care.

Caution, however, must be used to avoid coupling payments to compliance with unproven practices or driving blind compliance with guidelines, many of which are resented by providers who consider it an insult to be asked to practice cookbook medicine.

Without a systematic approach using innovative business and clinical design tools and modern process improvement methods, it is unlikely that significant changes in the reimbursement model, by themselves, can change the actual frontline delivery system from a predominantly volume-based production model to a more value-based production model.

Ideally, providers will develop new talents that allow them to map, design, measure, and truly understand their care processes. Most importantly, they will need to use bedside-derived outcomes data to refine those processes and spread this newfound knowledge to their colleagues to prompt improvements in care delivery. To do this, practitioners will have to become more adept at tasks such as Lean care process mapping, cost accounting (particularly with a technique known as time-driven, activity-based cost accounting) and data-driven performance improvement.[6]

SUMMARY

There is no doubt that the reimbursement system is moving inexorably toward more value-based contracting models. CMS, in particular, is taking bold strides in this direction through the MACRA/MIPS and APM models, the BPCI model, and its ACO or MSSP models. Commercial payers, as is usually the case, are following CMS's lead and creating value-based initiatives of their own. In response, many providers are now affiliating through entities such as CINs and ACOs (VBRAs) that allow them to operate successfully under these new agreements.

Reorganization under a new acronym, however, is not enough. Providers who join VBRAs must understand that the entity's primary mission must not be to merely contract for more dollars but to move the needle when it comes to creating higher value (quality and cost) for the patients cared for by the VBRAs participants. This often involves changing well-entrenched behaviors and practice patterns, which can be quite challenging. Furthermore, when there's money involved a lot of dissension or worsening of long-standing distrusts can make the task even harder to accomplish.

Nevertheless, this type of the value-based affiliation model of the future will be necessary for higher quality and lower costs within the healthcare system to indeed materialize. Hopefully, there will be steady progress in this area before draconian measures have to be used to ensure good outcomes at reasonable costs.

REFERENCES

1. Crosson FJ, Tollen LA. *Partners in Health: How Physicians and Hospitals Can Be Accountable Together.* San Francisco: Jossey-Bass; 2010.
2. Marren JP. "The FTC's Advocate Health Decision and Its Impact on PHOs, Clinical Integration, and Price Fixing." *The American Bar Association, Health Law Section,* June 2007.
3. Knight EM. "Bundled Payments: What are the Essentials You Need to Know." *www.CokerGroup.com.* January 2017. Accessed June 26, 2019. https://cokergroup.com/wp-content/uploads/2017/01/Bundled-Payment-What-are-the-Essentials-You-Need-to-Know_January-2017.pdf.
4. Knight EM. "Clinical Integration, The First Step Toward Value-based Healthcare Delivery." *Coker Group.* November 2018. Accessed June 26, 2019. https://cokergroup.com/wp-content/uploads/2019/02/Clinical_Integration_The_First_Step_in_Moving_Toward_Value-Based_Reimbursement_November_2018.pdf.
5. Leebenluft R, Weir T. Clinical Integration: Assessing the Antitrust Issues. In *Health Law Handbook, ed. A.D. Gosfield.* West Group, A Thomson Company; 2004.
6. Porter ME, Teisberg EO. *Redefining Health Care: Creating Value-based Competition on Results.* Boston: Harvard Business Review Press; 2006.

CHAPTER 13

Group Mergers

Many of the previous chapters have discussed options for provider practices seeking to affiliate with hospitals or health systems. Nevertheless, there are plenty of opportunities for providers to remain independent. While the number of solo practitioners has drastically declined in recent years due to the financial and operational pressures now keenly present in the industry, practices still have a unique opportunity to compete with healthcare organizations if they are of sufficient size. This "strength-in-numbers" concept is evident throughout the nation where conglomerates of healthcare providers—either of a single specialty or across an array of specialties—are becoming more prevalent. Further, as the industry continues to emphasize value, even going so far as site neutrality laws, these independent, merged organizations may be more competitive and successful than their aligned partners in some regards.

In this chapter, we outline the different types of mergers, critical considerations for merging, and the process itself.

SINGLE-SPECIALTY VS. MULTI-SPECIALTY MERGERS

One of the most common paths for mergers is combining practices of the same specialty to create instantaneous growth and market presence. As with all mergers, there also are key economies of scale to be realized when two once-competing practices merge their operations. Further, with a combined revenue stream, the practice may be able to afford the equipment, software, or staff that was once too costly to support.

The second type of merger is a multi-specialty merger in which providers come together under a single umbrella to offer myriad service offerings. Although this may require significantly more due diligence and likely will be more complicated and costly to initiate, it can have extremely high returns for the providers. These mergers typically are much larger than the single-specialty mergers and can often serve as a single point of care for patients, creating a more pleasing experience for the patient and provider. Thus, the practice can retain almost all revenue tied to a patient vs. referring out of the practice. If the practice also has significant ancillaries, this strategy can be highly profitable.

While these two types differ significantly in the post-merger operations, most of the considerations and processes are similar. Thus, unless otherwise stated, the following sections apply equally to both.

Types of Mergers

Both single-specialty and multi-specialty mergers typically fall into two major categories—legal or operational mergers—which differ based on the level of integration present. As with the other affiliation options, these differences can be extremely nuanced; hybrid structures are common as well.

Legal Merger

Under this scenario, a legal entity is created either through a NewCo or as Practice A merging with Practice B. Regardless, all groups and providers operate under one tax identification number (TIN), with operations remaining relatively the same as they were before the merger. Some administrative activities would merge (e.g., payer contracting, accounting, and the like), but parties combine very few, if any, clinical processes, or facilities. Further, parties would maintain a somewhat separate governance structure (though specific governance processes would be rolled up depending upon the newly created operating agreement). Figure 13.1 outlines the pros and cons of a legal merger.

FIGURE 13.1. Pros and Cons of a Legal Merger

PROs	CONs
• Has minimal impact on each group with respect for significant major operational changes • Has minimal impact on historical clinical functions/processes • Offers joint contracting opportunities • Provides group purchasing opportunities • Allows the possibility of economies of scale depending on the level of integration	• Has weak or limited economies of scale • Diminishes a collaborative mindset; typically, supports a *pod-like* mentality • Reduces the ability for clinical integration in the future

Full/Operational Merger

The full/operational merger is the opposite of the legal merger in that all operations, economics, and governance are consolidated within the NewCo. This consolidation includes standardization of virtually all functions across the practice to ensure a seamless patient care experience regardless of the location. Thus, ultimately, even the facilities are merged and/or consolidated so there is no distinction between the historical entities. Often, a legal or hybrid merger is a step toward the process of merging operationally and can serve as a compatibility test. Figure 13.2 details the pros and cons of a full/operational merger.

FIGURE 13.2. Pros and Cons of Full/Operational Merger

PROs	CONs
• Maximizes economies of scale • Provides streamlined efficiencies through consolidated operations • Increases ability to achieve the value proposition through enhanced care coordination functionalities	• May be arduous to implement • May entail significant changes to operational/clinical functions • Introduces potential cultural changes

Hybrid Legal/Full Merger

While hybrid structures do exist and may be hugely successful in specific scenarios, the legal or full merger structures are more common than hybrids. As the name suggests, the merged structure falls somewhere between the two types in the level of integration. The NewCo would be created, and the parties would agree to merge select operational functions while maintaining the other activities of their respective companies separately. Again, this avenue can be a stepping-stone toward a full merger, determining if the two parties will work well together culturally. See Figure 13.3 to review the pros and cons of a hybrid merger.

While the operations will vary based on the specific transaction under consideration, Figure 13.4 provides an example of how a merger may differ between a legal-only and full merger.

Note: Hybrid models of the two ends of more extreme structural scenarios are possible, if not probable and preferred. Therefore, certain features of both ends of the spectrum also are possible.

FIGURE 13.3. Pros and Cons of a Hybrid Merger

PROs	CONs
• Offers streamlined efficiencies through some consolidated operations • Has minimal impact on some of the more complex areas • Introduces limited cultural changes and implications for the current workflow • Provides the ability to customize the merged structure, as desired	• Does not fully utilize economies of scale • May entail operational challenges with oversight and monitoring with the merger of only some functions

FIGURE 13.4. Distinctions Between Legal-only and Full Merger

	Legal-Only Merger	Full Operational/MSO Merger
General Issues		
Tax ID Numbers	Each practice would operate under one TIN	Each practice would operate under one TIN
Physical Locations	Some consolidation over time	Consolidate geographic locales reasonably quickly—a major driver of the practices' proposed merger
Physician Employer	By unit or by a holding company	By centralized corporate entity
Governance	Centralized in certain areas, independent in others	Centralized
Operations		
Day-to-Day	Left at practice level; some centralization	Some decentralization; mostly centralized
Clinical	Mainly up to physician; some centralization	Still primarily up to each physician, but with more centralized decision making
Billing and Collections	Centralized; corporate office	Centralized; corporate office
Staffing/ Personnel	Employed by a holding company; decisions made at each location	Employed by central company; decisions largely centralized
Benefits	Centralized	Centralized

(Continued on next page)

FIGURE 13.4. Distinctions Between Legal-only and Full Merger *(continued)*

	Legal-Only Merger	Full Operational/MSO Merger
Accounting/ Finance	Centralized at the corporate office	Centralized at the corporate office
Strategic Issues		
Strategic Planning	Centralized with group input	Centralized with "board" input
Physician Comp/ IDP	Could be left individualized for each "site"	Largely one standard plan (at least over time)
Information Technology	Centralized	Centralized
Corporate Structure	Somewhat centralized; some individuality	Highly centralized; total merger
Ancillaries	Ability to expand; overall sharing	Ability to expand; overall sharing
Marketing	Mostly centralized, though, some based on practice/geographic location	Centralized, though could be targeted based on factors
Community Presentation	"Group" presentation; maintain some individuality	"Group" presentation
Measure Clinical Performance	High	High
Level of Autonomy	More than a full merger, less than current	None; corporate identity would be the primary goal
Realizing Economies of Scale	Medium to High	Highest

Reasons to Merge

In determining the go-forward strategy, it is important first to consider the "why" of the merger.

- What are the long-term goals?
- What issues are the parties attempting to mitigate?
- What does the practice want to provide the patient as an outcome of this merger?

The answers to these questions will inform (1) whether merging is a recommended approach, (2) what type of merger should be pursued (both in terms of pursuing a single-specialty or multi-specialty strategy and legal-only/operational/hybrid), and (3) the specific partner(s) to pursue. Though there are a host of reasons to merge, Figure 13.5 outlines a few key considerations.

FIGURE 13.5. Reasons to Merge

Economies of Scale	Risk-Spreading/ Management	Defensive Drivers
Market Growth/Reach	Survival/Critical Mass	Debt Capacity/Cash Acquisition
Flexibility/Market Strength	Financial Gain	Hospital Relations
Talent/Diversification	Accountable Care Era Strategy	Recruitment

The first part of the merger due diligence is to identify the reasons for merging, which should serve as the foundation for discussions going forward.

Merger Considerations

Mergers offer countless benefits; however, there also are several serious drawbacks for practices to consider before pursuing. As with any venture, they are costly in terms of both financial and human resources and require significant vetting to ensure success. Moreover, post-merger, there will be extensive changes (regardless of the type) and subsequent challenges. The parties should take the time to consider these obstacles before pursuing. Figure 13.6 presents a few of these issues to study throughout the process.

Merger Process

Overall, the merger typically is divided into three stages: Assessment, Merger Design, and Implementation.

Assessment

Typically, potential partners are identified (though not committed to a merger) and discussions commence with both parties. During this time, the fundamentals of the alliance are evaluated, with both parties outlining their levels of interest, the impetus for merging, and response to critical issues that may arise (e.g., merger type, equity buy-in, income

FIGURE 13.6. Challenging Issues to Consider with Mergers

Major Global Issues	Post-Merger Issues	Pre-Merger Issues
1. Structural 2. Operational 3. Relational 4. Governance 5. Financial 6. Physical and Facility 7. Clinical	1. Income Distribution Plan 2. Managed-Care Reimbursement 3. Costs and Economies of Scale 4. Operations and Marketing 5. Physician Supply, Recruitment, and Retention 6. Organizational Structure 7. Clinical Differences 8. Management/Administration 9. Staffing 10. Clinical Research Studies 11. Information Technology, Including PM and EHR 12. Fiscal and Economic 13. Physical (Facilities) 14. Ancillary Investments	1. Investment Commitment 2. Expected Return-on-Investment 3. Commitment to Common Mission/Vision 4. Support of Providers 5. "Dominance" of a Single Practice

distribution plans, governance, leadership, etc.). The parties then work to vet and determine alternatives for all identified issues. If the key concerns are insurmountable, or if during discussions the parties agree that there isn't a strong cultural fit, the merger should be delayed or called off entirely. Thus, this is the *go-or-no-go* point of the process.

Often, a third party is engaged during this time to ensure an efficient and comprehensive vetting process, digging into these key issues without creating tension. Depending on the number of physicians and/or practices involved, the process can range anywhere from 45 to 90 days to complete, which encompasses both on-site and off-site analyses. The third party may conduct a cursory review of practice data to identify any major issues; however, there has been no detailed due diligence nor sharing of any confidential between the parties. Instead, this portion of the process is more focused on qualitative factors and vetting key foundational issues.

Merger Design

Based on the critical issues identified in the assessment phase, the parties then determine the proposed terms of the agreement. This matter is accomplished via a series of negotiation meetings, again based on the foundation outlined in the assessment (i.e., driving toward the long-term goals of the parties and avoiding the "deal breakers"). Once the terms are identified, the parties start the comprehensive operational and financial due diligence to ensure the viability of the prospective structure.

After validating the basis for the agreement through the due diligence, the parties work in concert with legal counsel to draft the formal legal documents. These documents typically include an operating agreement for the new entity, as well as employment agreements for the providers. This activity includes the engagement of a qualified healthcare attorney to assist with this process to identify compliance risks and ensure the formation of a sound entity. Once these impediments are remedied, the implementation of the merger as outlined on paper begins.

The parties themselves can facilitate the merger process (likely driven by the administrative leadership) or they may engage a third-party advisor for this role. While completing the work through internal leaders may be the more cost-effective choice, hiring an independent expert may be a wiser choice. Using in-house leadership may be tenuous to complete the negotiations tactfully and swiftly as the parties have a bias toward their own practices. Thus, the parties typically will opt to continue working, with the third-party advisor engaged for the assessment and/or hire an alternative.

Implementation

Once the entity has been legally formed, the parties work to implement the agreed-upon structure. Again, this can be performed internally or supported by a third party. Based on the agreed strategy, this function may be accomplished by the newly hired or appointed leader of the practice.

Depending upon the merger, this process can take from six months to two years to accomplish. The providers/practices likely will be required during this time to take on some debt within the new entity or contribute capital to fund the operational development. Figure 13.7 provides a sample checklist, though by no means complete, of the activities involved in a merger.

FIGURE 13.7. Sample Merger Task List

Task	Responsible Party	Due Date	Status
1. Obtain bids for a bank account.			
2. Establish new TIN for the new entity.			
3. Develop capital expenditure plan for major purchases.			
4. Obtain financing based on capital expenditure plan.			
5. Contact payers to set up new contracts.			
6. Establish compensation model.			
7. Set up billing system/practice management system.			
8. Establish an accounting system.			
9. Establish payroll process.			
10. Identify and negotiate a lease assignment of existing leases.			
11. Establish an overall staffing plan.			
12. Obtain health and other insurance coverage plans for self and/or employees.			
13. Establish a pension/retirement plan for self and/or employees.			
14. Obtain malpractice coverage for the group.			
15. Establish relationships with medical supply vendors.			
16. Develop all associated human resources documentation.			
17. Purchase hardware that is compatible with new technologies.			
18. Notify state and local licensing boards of change of employment.			
19. Update all utilities and bills with the new entity.			
20. Create a conversion plan for patient information.			

(Continued on next page)

FIGURE 13.7. Sample Merger Task List *(continued)*

Task	Responsible Party	Due Date	Status
21. Inform patients of merger and develop a process for creating a seamless transition.			
22. Establish a marketing plan for the newly merged entity.			

SUMMARY

Successfully completing a merger (notably a full merger) is an involved process that should not be considered lightly. Done correctly, it can provide an alternative to hospital alignment while still drastically improving practice operations and finances. Further, as practices continue to determine ways to complete surgical procedures, provide ancillaries, and manage patients at a lower cost, these practices can compete directly with hospitals and health systems, especially for value-based reimbursement models. Merged entities likely will continue to increase in popularity for this reason, as their size will enable practices to meet these imperatives and continue realizing strong revenues.

Before pursuing a merger, practices should give due consideration to the potential drawbacks outlined above and fully vet their potential partners. If done at the beginning of the initiative, it can be a healthy and informative exercise and will create a more seamless transition. Additionally, this pre-planning will result in a more cost-effective merger by hashing out the key issues ahead of time versus addressing them in negotiations (and with the assistance of legal counsel). Thus, we recommend working with a third-party entity to complete the merger process as identified and set the new entity up for a long-term solution.

CHAPTER 14

Information Technology Due Diligence in Mergers

IT due diligence is a detailed evaluation of the technical side of an organization, including any technical products it leverages, manufactures, or is in the process of developing. Until recently, IT due diligence was not considered an essential component of the acquiring entity's overall due diligence analysis. However, in today's economy, information management is the currency that drives all businesses, including healthcare.

Before the IT due diligence process begins, the acquiring entity's leadership should have a clear understanding of the goal of the overall mergers and acquisitions transaction and how technology will play a part in its success. Often, the acquiring entity is looking to leverage its acquisition's technology and staff as part of its integration plan and support its ability to scale their operations. Conversely, the organization may decide to continue to manage the acquisition as a standalone entity with little to no integration planned.

IT due diligence is a critical exercise in an organization's investment cycle, whether it is an inpatient health system, private equity firm, investment bank, or acquiring physician practice. Understanding the purpose of information technology, including software, hardware, medical devices, etc., in the overall due diligence process is necessary to knowing how to target your analysis and ultimately maximize the investment of the assets being acquired. The strategy behind the IT due diligence determines what resources will be needed, where they will spend their time, and what questions must be answered so investors can make sound business decisions.

This chapter provides a brief introduction to some considerations that are relevant when preparing for an information technology disclosure or considering such disclosed information in the context of a mergers and acquisitions due diligence exercise.[1]

IT FACTORS TO CONSIDER

The information technology aspects of a due diligence analysis are basically the same as those for any other aspect of the due diligence process. Considerations around the structure of the proposed transaction could include, for example, a share purchase, an asset purchase, or a merger. The proposed construction of the deal will dictate to a great extent the various aspects of the information technology that require special attention under due diligence. For example, in the event a proposed transaction is an asset transfer, prohibitions or limitations on the assignment of software licenses will be relevant, while change control provisions will be relevant in the case of share purchases.[1]

Beyond the structure of the proposed transaction, it is important to understand in detail the information technology that will establish the subject matter of the due diligence review. More broadly, it will be necessary to obtain details of three specific areas:

- The information technology assets owned or used by the entity.
- Relevant documents supporting the information technology assets and third parties, including records related to service levels, technical and functional specifications, and warranties.
- The rights of and obligations to third parties in respect of those information technology assets.[2]

The complete disclosure of information technology resources and the role each asset plays in the entity's operations is critical. Having a full understanding of these assets will empower prospective buyers to determine how significant the technology and supporting vendor-partners are to the business operations and, consequently, the value of the proposed transaction.

For example, if a software asset such as an electronic health record (EHR) system provides the buyer with a competitive advantage or is a direct revenue driver, that asset will be valuable to the prospective buyer and in the due diligence review. The goal is to identify potential duplications in the information technology systems that the acquiring entity may wish to consider sunsetting or renegotiate contract terms during post-merger activities. With software assets, the typical information collected and evaluated is:

- An inventory of software used by the acquiring entity.

- Agreements related to the software assets, such as license, support, maintenance, service levels, escrow agreements.
- Documented policies and procedures, administrative and user manuals guides, and information on user access protocols.
- Active or planned co-development programs.

The hardware assets data collected include:

- Network and system diagrams of the hardware architecture.
- An inventory of hardware assets.
- Third-party agreements such as licenses, support, service level, and maintenance agreements, and disaster recovery and business continuity procedures.

Regarding hardware and software assets, contractual arrangements with third parties such as license agreements are important. These agreements highlight the rights and the scope of those rights the buyer may acquire through the proposed transaction. Licensing provisions may only be contained not in license agreements but also be part of various other initiatives, such as joint venture, consulting, development, and settlement agreements. If the acquiring entity is leveraging open-source software, the buyer is subject to the terms of an open-source software license agreement. Open-source and third-party software licenses may be an important factor in the proposed merger and acquisition (M&A) transaction, as they could dictate the terms on which the software can be licensed to third parties. Integration of open-sourced software and licensed software should be evaluated to determine its impact and future cost of integration into other parts of the business.

It also is essential to recognize that information technology is increasingly acquired as *software-as-a-service* or as part of a *cloud computing* strategy, which requires careful evaluation. Because of the extent to which information technology has become an integral part of how businesses operate and often a significant contributor to or source of competitive advantage, the appropriate review of information technology during a due diligence project is critical.[2]

In the approach to the due diligence, as established above, the focus is on a more *traditional* information technology environment.

IT DUE DILIGENCE PROCESS

IT due diligence traditionally begins following a sufficient assessment of the legal and financial aspects of merger and acquisition (M&A)

transaction. If the determination is that for legal or financial reasons a deal is not a viable option for moving forward, assessing the technology ecosystem would be useless. Technology should be considered an enabler to the business strategy and evaluated in the context of its application to that strategy.

If the assessment is positive, the team will gather as much external information as is readily available in the public sphere. Sources such as the organization's and vendors' websites, and social media should be explored to learn as much as possible about the acquiring entity and its senior leadership. Next, the IT due diligence team will reach out to the designated technical contact at the acquisition site and submit to them a Request for Information (RFI) document or comprehensive checklist of areas requiring evaluation.

Areas to evaluate during the due diligence process should include the following:

- IT and administrative staff
- Software and services utilized
- Hardware
- Network infrastructure
- Backup and recovery
- Network security
- IT strategic plan
- Cybersecurity
- Cloud-based services
- Contractual agreements
- Intellectual property
- IT policies and procedures
- Financial budgets
- Business associate agreements
- Vendors and third parties
- Audits results
- Software development process
- Products and services
- Confidentiality, non-compete, and non-solicitation agreements
- Intellectual property assignment agreements

In the sections below, we will explore in greater detail some of the items that require a thorough analysis.

IT and Administrative Staff

One of the first areas that should be evaluated is the staff capabilities of the organization being considered for acquisition. This inventory should include the name, title, department, location, supervising manager, industry certifications, key areas of responsibility, annual salary, start date, and full- or part-time status. An internal staff member on the due diligence team may be able to issue an alert if a key team member is disgruntled about the transition and might be exploring other job opportunities.

It is vital to have a good understanding of the strengths, weakness, and culture of the IT staff. This insight makes it possible to determine who will be a good fit once the two organizations begin to integrate resources. Additionally, this exercise will identify the remaining gaps the acquiring entity must address post-acquisition such as training and required certification, security, and system administration rights of staff. It will also encompass a determination of whether there is an expectation that a staff reduction will occur as part of the acquisition. The team's assessment can determine the real impact on operations if these reductions take place.

It is beneficial to include a person(s) from the acquired entity as part of the evaluation team to gather inside knowledge on staff capabilities and personalities, which can help the organization facilitate a smoother transition post-acquisition.

The team should also determine if the acquiring organization is experiencing a significant amount of attrition as part of the IT department's culture. Is there a high level of employee dissatisfaction in the department or low-performing team members? Finally, how satisfied is the staff with the support they now receive from the information systems department?

Network and System Infrastructure

Another objective of the IT due diligence is to identify potential cost savings from the anticipated consolidation of services and resources such as hosting, telecom, software licensing, hardware, and consulting services. Areas such as the transfer of software licensing and early termination of redundant services may involve unexpected costs. Do not assume that consolidation equates to immediate cost savings. The acquiring organization may take an initial financial hit as part of the integration strategy before realizing any savings or economies of scale post-acquisition.

Post-integration of IT services can take months and sometimes years. A post-integration plan should be developed after the deal is completed to set expectations and identify resource requirements to ensure its success. Some areas to consider as part of the technology integration plan are:

- Data center, network operations center, security operations center, etc.
- Phone system and network integration
- Email
- System integration
- Mobile and cloud-based platform
- Helpdesk and field support
- Key clinical and business applications

The IT due diligence team determines whether IT incurs any expenses for ongoing and/or planned technology initiatives. These expenditures include additional staff, consultants, and vendor professional services. The acquiring entity will have a better handle on the skills sets and staff they will need to retain or recruit, especially in areas where there may be a shortage of skilled IT professionals (e.g., cybersecurity). It is advantageous to be as proactive as possible and begin mapping out an integration strategy to ensure momentum is not lost post-merger.

Products and Services

As a part of the due diligence process, the team should compile an inventory and description of all software products and solutions acquired to include collecting the following information:

- Software name
- Description/purpose of software
- Departments that utilize the software
- How the software is delivered to the end-user (e.g., client/server, cloud, mobile, etc.)
- The number of licenses that are purchased and in use
- The current version in use

- Vendor support contacts
- Industry certifications
- The IT department administrators and technical support providers
- Whether the software is off-the-shelf, open-sourced, home-grown, or shareware

Often, there are a handful of key applications (e.g., EHR, claims, scheduling, financial, email, etc.) that most organization use, and it is crucial to gain as much insight about these systems as possible. These applications may offer the greatest opportunity for cost savings or, on the other hand, could continue to burden the organizations with additional overhead if they are not integrated successfully during post-acquisition.

The due diligence team also should survey the end-users to determine how satisfied they are with the use and support of these applications. The scalability of these systems that are in place should be assessed to increase the number of users or transactions flowing through the application.

Finally, it is critical to evaluate and inventory the system and/or administrative interfaces and the data migration strategy that will be needed. The questions include:

- What systems leverage the interface(s)?
- Who provides technical support?
- What IT users have control of the interface(s)?
- What data repositories are currently in place?
- How can the data be migrated from the current system into other platforms?

IT Strategic Plan

A review and evaluation of the current IT strategic plan is a necessary function of the IT due diligence team. The IT strategic plan provides a high-level roadmap that aligns the current and future technology investment with the organization's overall business priorities. The team will confirm whether the acquired entity has a plan. If it doesn't, they should be concerned that the organization they are considering purchasing is not proactive or lacks the necessary internal expertise to lead them through a series of technology transformation initiatives.

The IT strategic plan is a vital starting point for understanding the current state of affairs within the acquired entity. It also provides valued insight into additional items the team might not have considered as part of its initial assessment.

Hardware

Compiling an inventory of all purchased and leased hardware is a critical part of the due diligence process. The inventory includes the names, models, operating system, age, location, and current value of all the hardware. The inventory assessment should include but not be limited to the following:

- Desktops, laptops, and mobile devices
- Computer servers
- Routers, switches, firewalls
- Monitoring and recording devices
- Disk storage
- Phones
- Networked medical devices
- Printers, scanners, copiers, multifunction devices

During the assessment, the team should determine whether the systems have currently supported operating systems, firmware updates, maintenance, and lease agreements in place. If the acquiring entity plans to integrate the acquired company's technology into its portfolio, it is necessary to know whether the current technology is compatible with its own. If not, what will be the migration strategy from the legacy hardware into its own? How proficient is the acquired entity's IT staff in supporting their hardware? Overall, the IT due diligence must have a good understanding of the acquiring company's integration plan. Will they operate autonomously or assimilate into the standard corporate technology ecosystem? Another migration option is to allow entities to use a more ubiquitous platform that is cloud-based or PaaS/IaaS (Platform as a Service/Infrastructure as a Service) as a more cost-effective and scalable integration strategy.

Other hardware such as access cards, mobile hotspots, wireless cards, key fobs, and biomedical devices should be inventoried and evaluated for their potential to be integrated and supported post-acquisition.

Understanding the current and future hardware needs will provide executive leaders decisive insight into what will be required to provide ongoing support for the life cycle of the technology that is being acquired.

Server and Network Infrastructure

An accurate and complete network diagram that shows all entry points, servers, firewalls, LAN, and WAN connections is part of the due diligence process. The IT Department of the acquired company should be able to provide a comprehensive diagram that the due diligence team can use to evaluate a plan for integration post-acquisition.

It also is critical to gain an understanding of the current disaster recovery and business continuity strategy that must be supported and/or re-architected. In addition to reviewing a network topology diagram, the team should identify tools currently being used to monitor network traffic and bandwidth, CPU utilization, disk space, network, and endpoint security.

Finally, if the organization has its own server room/data center, technologies such as fire suppression, UPS (uninterruptable power supply), generator backup, and cooling, they must be evaluated to determine the capabilities for post-merger integration. If cloud services are used, the team needs to investigate where the data is stored and backed up. Many managed service providers (MSPs) leverage data centers and network infrastructure around the world. They must meet all regulatory standards or pinpoint the specific environment if the data are stored in one location. Most MSPs will allow an organization to assign the data to a specific facility that delivers disaster recovery and business continuity service in an alternate geographical location.

If the acquiring company is leveraging a PaaS/IaaS solution from the MSP, the team must know what is required technically to migrate systems and data from that environment to another, if necessary. Lastly, due diligence should reveal the cost to scale up current IT investments as part of the post-acquisition integration plan.

Backup and Recovery

Disaster recovery (DR) and business continuity (BC) are necessary to the survival of all business operations in this electronic data-driven environment. Every due diligence exercise should include an evaluation of the acquired entity's DR and/or BC plan. IT disaster recovery is generally one component of an overall BC plan that covers all business operations.

It is important first to validate that a DR/BC plan exists. If a reliable and executable plan is not in place, this gap could signal a significant unbudgeted expense to the acquisition. Also, the lack of a plan would put the organization at risk post-acquisition in the event of a natural or manmade disaster. It is not only important to confirm a plan has been developed, it is equally significant to confirm it is evaluated periodically, at least annually. If there is no IT DR/BS plan in place, this should raise a flag as to the credibility of the current IT team. System backups should be evaluated and restored regularly. Tabletop or simulated disaster scenarios should be conducted at least annually, and all critical systems should be restored periodically.

The due diligence team should evaluate whether any additional expense will be incurred to integrate the acquisition in the current environment. For example, will there be a need for extra storage, bandwidth, hardware, vendor services, and the like to ensure the BC of the recently acquired assets? Is the newly migrated IT staff trained and experienced in the organization's DR/BC protocols and processes?

Network and Cybersecurity

In March 2019, healthcare data breaches continued to be reported at a rate of one per day. Thirty-one healthcare data breaches were reported to the Department of Health and Human Services' (HHS) Office for Civil Rights by HIPAA-covered entities and their business associates. The March 2019 total is almost 14% higher than the average of the past 60 months.[3]

Network security breaches are on the rise and cybersecurity now is one of the top issues of healthcare executives.[4] As a part of the IT due diligence deliverables, it is necessary to evaluate the acquired company's network security strategy and technology investment. Software and hardware manufacturers regularly release updates and patches to address vulnerabilities in their solutions. An explanation of how the acquired entity stays current with all vendor security updates and patches is needed. Due diligence should include a request and evaluation of a documented process for deploying antivirus, patch match management of workstations, laptops, servers, network (i.e., firewalls, routers, etc.), intrusion detection, and mobile devices.

Other Internet of Things (IoT) devices that can connect to the acquired entity's network can pose as much of a security risk as traditional technology platforms. Networked medical devices, video conferencing solutions, security cameras, climate control systems, and consumer-owned devices are just a few potential entry points for cybercriminals. If the acquiring entity plans to integrate its acquisition's infrastructure into their corporate network, they must determine if the necessary technical expertise is currently in place to effectively manage all aspects of the new entity's cybersecurity environment. They also will have to evaluate whether it will be necessary to invest capital in updating or enhancing post-acquisition infrastructure to mitigate the risk of data breaches.

Network and cybersecurity are not limited to hardware and software protections. Insider threats should be evaluated and processes/procedures realigned when needed. A review of end-user cybersecurity training, password policies, email, and web browsing best practices, etc., should be considered during the IT due diligence evaluation. The assessment should also include background checks of staff, review of business associate agreements, phishing, social engineering, and penetration testing initiatives.

Information is the most valuable currency an organization has in today's digital commerce economy. The IT due diligence team, therefore, should pay special attention to this part of the evaluation process.

Agreements

The terms and conditions in an organization's contractual agreements are other elements the team should evaluate as a part of the due diligence exercise. The process calls for close attention to highlight any penalties for early cancellation of services, automatic renewal options, service level agreements, time and material fees, indemnification clauses, nonsupported services, hours of support, and data migration fees.

Although these issues should surface during the legal due diligence process, it is always a good practice to have the IT team review and provide commentary on any currently executed IT-related contracts.

In their investigation, the team may determine that an agreement is inadequate or, in some cases, does not exist. The acquiring entity will need to consider these matters in terms of the cost of entering into a new agreement or adding them to an existing contract.

Data Backup, Recovery, and Business Continuity

Data backup and recovery should be an integral part of the BC plan and information technology DR plan, advises the official website of the Department of Homeland Security. Developing a data backup strategy begins with identifying what data to backup, selecting and implementing hardware and software backup procedures, scheduling and conducting backups, and periodically validating that data has been accurately backed up.

During the due diligence process, a BC plan helps ensure the business processes will continue during a time of emergency or disaster, according to Techopedia.[6] Such emergencies or disasters might include an act of nature, such as fires, snowstorms, floods, etc., or any other case where business activity is unable to occur under normal conditions. The acquiring entity needs to make sure that a BC plan is in place, and it highlights all such potential threats. The acquiring party should devise a plan to ensure continued operations should the risk become a reality.

Specifically, the BC plan involves the following:

- Analysis of organizational threats
- A list of the primary tasks required to keep the organization's operations flowing
- Management contact information that is easy to locate
- Explanation of where personnel should go if there is a disastrous event
- Information on data backups and organization site backup
- Collaboration among all facets of the organization
- Buy-in from everyone in the organization[5]

If a plan does not exist, the cost to address issues that impact operations could be steep. Finally, you should confirm that the plan is evaluated routinely (at least annually). Testing identifies potential gaps in the plan and evaluates its practicality in real-world situations.

IT due diligence in healthcare involves special considerations related to data privacy and security. Any significant interruption to business operations can have a detrimental impact on patient care. A thorough and detailed assessment of an organization IT infrastructure, policies, procedures, staff, and vendor relationships is critical. Protected Health Information (PHI) includes demographic and clinical information that is related to the delivery of care or billing for medical services used to identify an individual. It also requires a deep dive into technologies related to the HIPAA Privacy and Security Rule and the resources necessary to remain in compliance.

SUMMARY

Until recently, IT was not considered to be an essential component of the acquiring entity's overall due diligence analysis. However, in today's economy, information management is the currency that drives all businesses, including healthcare and IT due diligence is a critical exercise in an organization's investment cycle for all parties involved.

The importance of understanding the appropriate purpose of information technology, including software, hardware, medical devices, etc., in overall due diligence process is in knowing how to target analysis and ultimately maximize the investment of the acquired assets. The strategy behind the IT due diligence identifies required resources, shows where time will be invested, and asks the questions that need to be answered so investors can make sound business decisions.

This chapter addressed considerations relevant to preparing for an information technology disclosure or considering such disclosed information in the context of an M&A due diligence exercise.

REFERENCES

1. Steyn W. Due Diligence in M&A Transactions: Information Technology Considerations. Al Tamimi & Co. December 2011. https://www.tamimi.com/law-update-articles/due-diligence-in-ma-transactions-information-technology-considerations. Accessed October 10, 2019.
2. "March 2019 Healthcare Data Breach Report." *HIPAA Journal.* April 15, 2019. https://www.hipaajournal.com/march-2019-healthcare-data-breach-report. Accessed August 13, 2019.

3. Stewart A. The Top 10 Challenges Healthcare Executives Anticipate for 2019. *Becker's ASC Review*. September 25, 2018. https://www.beckersasc.com/leadership-management/the-top-10-challenges-healthcare-executives-anticipate-for-2019.html. Accessed August 13, 2019.
4. Ready, IT Disaster Recovery Plan. https://www.ready.gov/business/implementation/IT. Accessed October 10, 2019.
5. What is a Business Continuity Plan (BCP)? - Definition ....Technopedia. https://www.techopedia.com/definition/3/business-continuity-plan-bcp. Accessed October 10, 2019.

CHAPTER 15

Legal and Regulatory Considerations

This chapter provides an overview of the legal aspects of affiliation options that are available to physicians in the structures described in the book. The affiliation models will be addressed, including physician employment, professional services agreements, joint equity ventures, private equity transactions, private equity-like transactions, clinical co-management, CINs, and various forms of merger.

Certain legal rules apply to all these models, across the board. Others have more unique legal requirements, such as clinical co-management that has been described primarily in Advisory Opinions of the Office of Inspector General.

The focal point of the pertinent laws is squarely on physician compensation in each of the affiliation arrangements.

PHYSICIAN EMPLOYMENT AND PROFESSIONAL SERVICES AGREEMENTS

As is described in other parts of this book, physician employment and professional services agreements are a popular way for physicians to affiliate with health systems, hospitals, private equity firms, and with each other. Each of these arrangements includes physician compensation provisions that must be legally compliant. The basis for physician compensation may be determined by such factors as gross revenue, net cash collections, Relative Value Units or RVUs, tiered RVUs, bonuses, and other systems of allocation of revenue and expenses.

Most physician compensation systems involve both a fixed base salary and an additional bonus component; however, the foundation for most physician compensation is based on physician productivity measured by RVUs. (Note: Relative Value Units (RVUs) is a standard set by Medicare to determine the amount to pay doctors depending on their productivity. It is a number that defines the volume of work doctors perform when treating patients for all procedures and services covered under the **Physician Fee Schedule**. See https://www.cms.gov/medicare/medicare-fee-for-service-payment/physicianfeesched.)

THE LEGAL BASIS FOR RVUs

Federal law includes numerous references to RVUs. CMS has codified RVUs in the Code of Federal Regulations (CFR) at 42 CFR 414.22. These sections of the CFR describe in detail how to calculate RVUs. CMS also updates RVUs annually as part of the Medicare Physician Fee Schedule rulemaking process. In addition, RVU-based compensation is explicitly recognized in the Stark Law, where productivity bonuses based on RVUs are approved as an appropriate and lawful method to compensate physicians. See 42 CFR 411.352(i)(3)(i) "Special Rule for productivity bonuses and profit shares." This rule allows the payment of productivity bonuses based on services performed personally by the physician or services incident to those personally performed services.

Following are numerous legal considerations that impact physician compensation including RVU compensation systems:

1. Federal Stark Law 42 U.S.C. 1395nn
2. Federal Anti-Kickback Law 42 U.S.C. 1320a-7b(b)
3. Federal Advisory Opinions from the Office of the Inspector General
4. Federal tax law
5. State anti-kickback statutes
6. State corporate practice of medicine statutes
7. The Federal False Claims Act 31 U.S.C. 3729
8. The Medicare prohibition against assignment of receivables

The list above is not exhaustive and the regulations that have been promulgated under the laws above number in the thousands of pages. Each of these areas of law can have an impact on physician compensation. Please note that the Medicaid system provides no guidance in this regard and appears to rely on Medicare.

THE STARK LAW

Among the numerous laws that impact physician compensation, the Stark Law is the most restrictive and also the most punitive. The good news is that if a compensation arrangement meets the requirements of the Stark Law or one of its exceptions, in many cases the requirements of the other laws listed above also will be met. The bad news is that all physician compensation arrangements must comply with the Stark Law or one of its exceptions. There is little wiggle room and little room for interpretation. Further, failure to comply exposes the parties to heavy fines and penalties.

At the most basic level, the Stark Law prohibits a physician from referring a designated health service (DHS) to an entity if the physician has a direct or indirect financial relationship with that entity unless a specific exception applies. Under Stark, all physician compensation arrangements in all affiliations is defined as a financial relationship. Each of the exceptions is specifically worded and must be strictly complied with. Further, even practitioners who do not provide a significant volume of Medicare services must comply with the Stark Law if they participate in Medicare at all.

The Stark Law technically does not cover those elements of the physician's practice that are outside of Medicare or are not related to designated health services. However, it is rare for an organization to maintain two separate billing systems and two separate recordkeeping systems, with one for complying with Stark and one for a different compensation system that is not Stark compliant. The result is that virtually every physician compensation arrangement comes within the coverage of the Stark Law for practical or legal reasons.

The consequences of entering a financial arrangement that does not comply with the Stark Law or one of the exceptions can be harsh. As a baseline requirement, the involved parties must repay Medicare for any claims for DHS referrals made while the noncompliant arrangement was in place. Further, prohibited referrals made during the noncompliant arrangement may result in substantial fines and penalties.

While Stark violations typically do not involve a jail sentence, the civil penalties can be significant. For example, CMS may impose a fine of up to $15,000 per claim, regardless of the amount of the claim, be it $1 or $10,000. When those $15,000 fines are multiplied by the thousands of claims for DHS that may submitted based on referrals by a physician during a tainted arrangement, the fines can become astronomical, amounting to tens or even hundreds of millions of dollars in cases where the reimbursements from Medicare and revenue generated for the physician are comparatively small.

Finally, in serious cases, providers may be excluded from the Medicare program. This is a severe consequence given that few medical practitioners, hospitals, or facilities can survive without participation in the Medicare program.

EXCEPTIONS TO THE STARK LAW

While physician compensation in affiliation arrangements generally qualifies as a financial relationship governed and prohibited by the Stark Law, there are two principal exceptions: (1) the bona fide employment exception for W-2 employees; and (2) the personal services arrangement exception for independent contractors. Also, productivity bonuses utilizing RVUs are an explicitly recognized exception under Stark.

To understand how the exceptions work, it is necessary to understand definitions under the Stark Law:

1. **Physician.** The definition of physician includes a variety of practitioners including doctors of medicine, osteopathy, dentists, podiatrists, optometrists, and chiropractors.
2. **Designated Health Services.** The statute includes a list of services that are considered DHS. CMS annually updates and publishes in the Federal Register a detailed DHS list that uses CPT codes to more precisely define these terms. The DHS list is as follows:
   a. Clinical laboratory services
   b. Physical therapy services
   c. Occupational therapy services
   d. Radiology services including MRI, CT, and ultrasound
   e. Radiation therapy services and supplies
   f. Durable medical equipment and supplies
   g. Parenteral and enteral nutrients, equipment, and supplies
   h. Prosthetics, orthotics, prosthetic devices, and supplies
   i. Home health services

j. Outpatient prescription drugs
k. Inpatient and outpatient hospital services.

Notably, professional services provided in a physician's office are not on the list, nor are surgeries and ambulatory surgery centers. The DHS list is broad and is updated in January of each year.

3. **Financial Relationship.** A financial relationship under Stark can be a direct or indirect ownership or investment interest, or a direct or indirect compensation arrangement, between a physician and an entity that furnishes DHS. This covers salary, bonuses, income guarantees, medical director payments, and on-call fees, in any form including RVUs. Further, financial relationships are construed broadly to include such relationships between DHS entities and physicians' immediate family members such as spouses, parents, children, siblings, and even more distant relations like stepparents, stepchildren, stepsiblings, in-laws, grandparents, and grandchildren and their spouses.

All compensation to physicians pursuant to affiliation arrangements including hospital employment is covered by Stark because employment establishes a financial relationship, and physicians typically refer to their employer hospital.

In contrast, to the extent that physician compensation in a medical group does not involve anything that is on the DHS list, that compensation is free of the restrictions of the Stark Law. However, once an affiliation relationship is established and a physician refers a DHS list item, it is covered by Stark. As a result of the pervasive coverage of the DHS list, most affiliation arrangements will need to structure the compensation in strict compliance with Stark.

STARK EXCEPTION FOR BONA FIDE EMPLOYMENT RELATIONSHIPS

The Stark Law does provide an exception for bona fide employment relationships. This covers any amount paid by an employer to a physician (or an immediate family member of such physician) who has a bona fide employment relationship with the employer for the provision of services if:

1. The employment is for identifiable services.
2. The amount of the compensation is:
   a. Consistent with the fair market value of the services; and
   b. Not determined in a manner that considers (directly or indirectly) the volume or value of any referrals by the referring physician.
3. The compensation is provided pursuant to an agreement that would be commercially reasonable even if no referrals were made to the employer.

The key point of the above is that the compensation in all affiliation arrangements must be fair market value. Fair market value is discussed in detail below.

STARK EXCEPTION FOR PERSONAL SERVICE ARRANGEMENTS

A Stark exception also is made for personal service arrangements in affiliation arrangements that involve someone who is not a W-2 employee. Affiliation arrangements including clinical co-management, CINs, medical director or on-call arrangements, and others involve payments of compensation to physicians who are not W-2 employees. The requirements of these arrangements are as follows:

1. The arrangement is set out in writing, signed by the parties, and specifies the services covered by the arrangement;
2. The arrangement covers all the services to be provided by the physician (or an immediate family member of such physician) to the entity;
3. The aggregate services contracted for do not exceed those that are reasonable and necessary for the legitimate business purposes of the arrangement;
4. The term of the arrangement is for at least 1 year;
5. The compensation to be paid over the term of the arrangement is:
   a. Set in advance,
   b. Does not exceed fair market value, and
   c. Is not determined in a manner that considers the volume or value of any referrals or other business generated between the parties; and

6. The services to be performed under the arrangement do not involve the counseling or promotion or a business arrangement or other activity that violates any state or federal law.

STARK DEFINITION FOR FAIR MARKET VALUE

The definition of fair market value under Stark affects almost every form of affiliation. The term "fair market value" means the value in arm's-length transactions, consistent with the general market value. "General market value" means the price that an asset would bring as the result of bona fide bargaining between well-informed buyers (health systems) and sellers (physicians) who are not otherwise in a position to generate business for the other party, or the compensation that would be included in a service agreement as the result of bona fide bargaining between well-informed parties to the agreement who are not otherwise in a position to generate business for the other party, at the time of the service agreement.

Usually, the fair market price is the compensation that has been included in bona fide service agreements with comparable terms at the time of the agreement, where the compensation has not been determined in any manner that takes into account the volume or value of anticipated or actual referrals.

DEFINITION OF GROUP PRACTICE

Many affiliation arrangements, including group mergers, physician employment, professional services agreements, and private equity transactions, will result in the physicians becoming part of a larger group practice that is part of a health system or associated with a platform entity owned by a private equity firm. When meeting a Stark exception, it is important to ensure that the arrangement meets the definition of Group Practice. As discussed further below, group practices may avail themselves of certain rules regarding the allocation of overall profits and productivity bonuses.

The term "group practice" means a group of two or more physicians legally organized as a partnership, professional corporation, foundation, not-for-profit corporation, faculty practice plan, or similar association:

1. In which each physician who is a member of the group provides substantially the full range of services which the physician routinely provides, including medical care, consultation, diagnosis, or treatment, through the joint use of shared office space, facilities, equipment, and personnel;
2. For which substantially all the services of the physicians who are members of the group are provided through the group and are billed under a billing number assigned to the group and amounts so received are treated as receipts of the group;
3. In which the overhead expenses of and the income from the practice are distributed in accordance with methods previously determined;
4. In which no physician who is a member of the group directly or indirectly receives compensation based on the volume or value of referrals by the physician;
5. In which members of the group personally conduct no less than 75 percent of the physician-patient encounters of the group practice; and
6. Which meets such other standards as the Secretary may impose by regulation.

SPECIAL RULE FOR PROFIT SHARES AND PRODUCTIVITY BONUSES IN GROUP PRACTICES

Since most affiliation arrangements include physician compensation involving base pay and bonus arrangements, it often is helpful to use special rules for bonuses that exist under Stark.

A physician in a group practice may be paid a bonus that is a share of "overall profits" of the group, provided that the share is not determined in any manner that is directly related to the volume or value of referrals of DHS by the physician.

Additionally, a physician in the group practice may be paid a productivity bonus based on services that he or she has personally performed, or services "incident to" such personally performed services, or both, provided that the bonus is not determined in any manner that is directly related to the volume or value of referrals of DHS by the physician.

"Overall profits" are the group's entire profits derived from DHS payable by Medicare or Medicaid or the profits derived from DHS payable by Medicare or Medicaid of any component of the group practice that consists of at least five physicians. Overall profits should be allocated in a reasonable and verifiable manner that is not directly related to the volume or value of the physician's referrals of DHS. The share of overall profits will be deemed not to relate directly to the volume or value of referrals if one of the following conditions is met:

1. The group's profits are divided per capita (for example, per member of the group or per physician in the group); or
2. Revenues derived from DHS are distributed based on the distribution of the group practice's revenues attributed to services that are not DHS payable by any federal healthcare program or private payer; or
3. Revenues derived from DHS constitute less than 5% of the group practice's total revenues, and the allocated portion of those revenues to each physician in the group practice constitutes 5% or less of his or her total compensation from the group.

In all affiliation arrangements, a productivity bonus must be calculated in a reasonable and verifiable manner that is not directly related to the volume or value of the physician's referrals of DHS. A productivity bonus will be deemed not to relate directly to the volume or value of referrals of DHS if one of the following conditions is met:

1. The bonus is based on the physician's total patient encounters or RVUs; or
2. The bonus is based on the allocation of the physician's compensation attributable to services that are not DHS payable by a federal health care program or private payer; or
3. Revenues derived from DHS are less than 5% of the group practice's total revenues, and the allocated portion of those revenues to each physician in the group practice constitutes 5% or less of his or her total compensation from the group practice.

Every party in an affiliation arrangement with physicians or medical groups must maintain thorough documentation of the systems, calculations, and processes that are used to determine physician compensation.

SPECIAL RULES ON COMPENSATION

In setting physician compensation, all affiliation arrangements should be aware of the following special rules that apply for purposes of the Stark exceptions discussed above:

1. Compensation is considered "set in advance" if the aggregate compensation, a time-based or per-unit of service-based (whether per-use or per-service) amount, or a specific formula for calculating the compensation is set in an agreement between the parties before the furnishing of the items or services for which the compensation is to be paid. The formula for determining the compensation must be set forth in sufficient detail so that it can be objectively verified, and the formula may not be changed or modified during the course of the agreement in any manner that takes into account the volume or value of referrals or other business generated by the referring physician.
2. Unit-based compensation (including time-based or per-unit of service-based compensation) is deemed not to take into account "the volume or value of referrals" if the compensation is fair market value for services or items actually provided and does not vary during the course of the compensation arrangement in any manner that takes into account referrals of DHS.
3. Unit-based compensation (including time-based or per-unit of service-based compensation) is deemed not to take into account "other business generated between the parties," provided that the compensation is fair market value for items and services actually provided and does not vary during the course of the compensation arrangement in any manner that takes into account referrals or other business generated by the referring physician, including private pay health care business (except for services personally performed by the referring physician, which are not considered "other business generated" by the referring physician).

"PER-CLICK" OR PERCENTAGE-BASED COMPENSATION

CMS has prohibited the use of per-service (per-click) and percentage-based compensation arrangements in lease agreements between physicians and DHS entities for equipment or office space. Under per-click arrangements, the lessee compensates the lessor for use of the space or equipment based on the number of services performed using the space or equipment. Similarly, under a percentage-based arrangement, the lessee pays the lessor a percentage of revenues generated from using the space or equipment. CMS, through rulemaking, has determined that such arrangements vary based on the volume or value of referrals and are illegal.

While per-click and percentage-based arrangements are expressly prohibited for office and equipment leases, they may be allowable with respect to other compensation arrangements. However, parties must take extra care to base such variable compensation on lawful elements of the arrangement—such as services actually performed by the physicians—and not on referrals. For example, CMS has indicated that physicians may be compensated per service or based on a percentage of revenues or collections for services they have personally performed. However, CMS has expressed skepticism about this approach in other arrangements, such as compensation for billing and collections service.

In general, per-click and percentage-based arrangements are allowable if they otherwise meet the requirements of a Stark exception, including the special rules on compensation discussed in the prior section.

LIMITING REFERRALS AND KEEPING REFERRALS WITHIN A NETWORK

The Stark Law does, in certain circumstances, allow a financial arrangement between a physician and a DHS entity to be conditioned on referrals to a specific entity. Specifically, a physician's compensation under an affiliation arrangement or from a bona fide employer or under a managed-care contract or other contract for personal services may be conditioned on the physician's referrals to a particular affiliate, provider, practitioner, or supplier, as long as the compensation arrangement strictly meets all of the following conditions:

1. Is set in advance for the term of the agreement;
2. Is consistent with fair market value for services performed and the payment does not consider the volume or value of anticipated or required referrals; and
3. Complies with both of the following conditions:

   a. The requirement to make referrals to a particular provider, practitioner, or supplier is set forth in a written agreement signed by the parties; and
   b. The requirement to make referrals to a particular provider, practitioner, or supplier ***does not apply*** if
      i. the patient expresses a preference for a different provider, practitioner, or supplier;
      ii. the patient's insurer determines the provider, practitioner, or supplier; or
      iii. the referral is not in the patient's best medical interests in the physician's judgment.
4. The required referrals relate solely to the physician's services covered by the scope of the affiliation agreement or employment or the contract, and the referral requirement is reasonably necessary to effectuate the legitimate business purposes of the compensation arrangement. In no event may the physician be required to make referrals that relate to services that are not provided by the physician under the scope of his or her employment or contract.

In summary, the requirements of the Stark Law that apply to compensation arrangements of physicians in any kind of affiliation arrangement are numerous and very complex. It is necessary to meet all applicable requirements under the Stark Law.

THE ANTI-KICKBACK STATUTE

The Anti-Kickback Statute (AKS) prohibits knowing or willful payments of any kind or inducement in return for referrals. To avoid being charged with a violation of the AKS, it is necessary to ensure payments are not made with the intent to induce referrals nor with the intent to limit medically necessary services for patients. Safe harbors provide guidance on how to establish protected and legally safe affiliation arrangements.

The most frequently used safe harbor in affiliation arrangements is known generally as the "personal services and the management contracts" safe harbor, which requires that the physician compensation agreement meet seven standards:

1. The agreement must be in writing;

2. The agreement must describe all the services to be provided;
3. If the agreement is periodic, sporadic, or part-time, it must precisely specify the schedule of the intervals;
4. The agreement must be for not less than one year;
5. Compensation must be set in advance, consistent with fair market value, and not determined in a manner that takes into account the volume or value of referrals;
6. The arrangement cannot involve the counseling or promotion of a business that violates state or federal law, and
7. The aggregate services do not exceed those reasonably necessary to accomplish the commercially reasonable purposes of the agreement.

Determining what is set in advance, fair market value, and commercially reasonable are the most difficult aspects of the agreements. The requirement that the compensation be set in advance is probably the one that is most often missed. Typically, it is necessary to engage a third-party valuation organization to review and comment upon the terms of the compensation agreement in order to ensure that the agreement meets these requirements. A good rule of thumb is that if the Stark exceptions are met, the compensation arrangement will meet the Anti-Kickback safe harbor.

NOT-FOR-PROFIT TAX RULES

If a not-for-profit hospital is the employer or the party to a merger or clinical co-management arrangement, additional rules apply. It is illegal to allow tax-exempt dollars to be paid to taxable individual physicians unless the payment is justified by the delivery of services of equal value. Inappropriate payments of this type are called "private inurement." Those services may be compensated only at fair market value, which should be determined by an independent third party or by comparison to an independent compensation survey. If private inurement or private benefit occurs, the hospital risks losing its tax-exempt status.

After a compensation system has been established, the compensation structure must be reviewed by an independent third-party valuation consultant. Or, at the very least, it must be compared to a valuation survey to verify that the compensation system results in overall compensation that is competitive and within the ranges of compensation paid to other similar practitioners. Again, these rules apply to any form of affiliation that involves a not-for-profit or tax-exempt organization.

CREDENTIALING

Economic credentialing systems can be linked to compensation systems in many affiliation arrangements. Hospitals use economic credentialing for physician profiling and loyalty determinations. To the extent that a physician scores poorly in the performance metrics used to determine compensation, a hospital that does economic credentialing can use the statistics against a practitioner. In the most egregious situations, physicians can lose privileges, or be expelled from CINs for failure to meet performance metrics.

Economic credentialing has been frequently challenged in lawsuits. However, hospitals have justified the practice in most cases in states where it is not prohibited by law.

THE MEDICARE ACCESS AND CHIP REAUTHORIZATION ACT

One of the recent developments with significant impact on physician compensation in many affiliation arrangements is the Medicare Access and CHIP Reauthorization Act (MACRA). MACRA changes the way Medicare pays for professional services provided by physicians and non-physician practitioners. Beginning in 2019, physicians are paid under one of two tracks: the Merit-Based Incentive Payment System (MIPS) or advanced alternative payment models (APMs). Medicare will continue to use the RVU-based fees established in the Physician Fee Schedule (PFS) to compensate physicians. However, the actual payments received by a physician will, in many cases, be adjusted to reflect penalties or bonuses earned by the physician. The specific adjustment will be based on the track in which the physician participates.

Most physicians will be paid under the MIPS, which is the default payment track. Under MIPS, physicians will be evaluated on their performance in four categories: quality, cost, practice improvement activities, and advancing care information (i.e., meaningful use of electronic health records [EHR]). Each physician will receive a score, which will be compared to a threshold score calculated annually by CMS. Physicians above the threshold score will receive a bonus payment; those below the threshold score will receive a negative adjustment. Physicians will be evaluated two years prior to applicable payments, which means that for 2019 payments, CMS will evaluate physician performance in 2017. The potential payment adjustments increase over time, from ±4% in 2019 to ±9% in 2021 and beyond.

In contrast, physicians who participate in certain APMs will not be subject to MIPS requirements and payment adjustments; instead, qualifying physicians, known as "qualifying participants" (QPs), will receive a lump-sum bonus payment of 5% of their revenues paid under the PFS each year, from 2019 through 2024. To become QPs, physicians must provide a certain, significant percentage of their services through a qualified advanced APM. To qualify as an advanced APM, a payment model must show use of a certified EHR, tie an amount of payment to quality metrics, and demonstrate providers taking on downside risk.

DHS entities that contract with physicians in all forms of affiliation models must consider how the potential positive and negative payment adjustments will affect those contracts, particularly in light of fair market value as discussed above. Significantly, the MACRA does not include any waiver of the Stark or Anti-Kickback laws. Therefore, physician compensation arrangements that attempt to address or incorporate the MACRA payment adjustments still must comply with those laws, including any applicable exceptions or safe harbors.

ADVISORY OPINIONS AND AFFILIATION MODELS

Affiliation models including PSAs, joint ventures, clinical co-management, and CINs, can obtain more guidance about proper structures and compensation from Advisory Opinions (AOs) issued by the Office of Inspector General (OIG). Three of these opinions are particularly relevant: AO 08-16, AO 11-15, and AO 12-22. (AO 08-16 means that it was the 8th opinion issued by the OIG in 2016).

- AO 08-16 addresses a "quality enhancement professional services agreement" between a hospital and a physician entity. While the arrangement presents some risk, the OIG found that sufficient safeguards were put in place to allow the system of base pay and bonuses for achieving "Pay for Performance" targets.

- AO 11-15 addresses a management services contract between a path lab and a physician-owned LLC and found the arrangement presents unacceptably high risk of illegal remuneration for the physicians involved.
- AO 12-22 addresses clinical co-management and found an acceptable arrangement involving fair market value payments of base compensation and bonus compensation for achieving performance metrics that were set in advance.

While these Advisory Opinions are expressly limited to their specific facts and not intended to serve as precedent, they do provide excellent guidance regarding what the OIG thinks about certain compensation arrangements. In fact, there is not a great deal of specific information about these arrangements that appears elsewhere in the law.

ANALYSIS OF AFFILIATION MODELS

Limited Affiliations

Limited models including arrangements for recruitment assistance, medical directorships, and call coverage must meet all the requirements stated above under Stark and Anti-Kickback. Because a Stark exception must be met, it is best to meet all requirements of an Anti-Kickback safe harbor.

Moderate Affiliations

Moderate affiliation including joint ventures, service line management, management services organizations and/or clinical co-management should follow the guidance that appears in the Advisory Opinions cited above. A close reading of these Advisory Opinions will provide an excellent example of the correct way to structure service line and co-management compensation arrangements with physicians.

Full Affiliations

Full integration involving private equity or health system acquisitions, merged groups, employment, professional services arrangements, and

CINs are clearly within the purview of Stark and Anti-Kickback. It is crucial to meet the requirements of these laws as described in their defined terms, structures of compensation requirements, fair market value, and commercially reasonable compensation requirements, incentives tied to performance, and others.

SUMMARY

Affiliation models offer great opportunity, but they carry with them a degree of risk presented by failing to meet the requirements of the applicable laws. That said, compensation systems that meet the Stark Law exceptions or that are within the Anti-Kickback safe harbors are a recognized as being lawful. It is best to make sure that in every affiliation arrangement, compensation is fair market value, commercially reasonable, and set in advance in a written agreement of one year or more.

CHAPTER 16

Options for Capital Procurement

Capital procurement is the source of funds used to meet required expenditures when consummating a transaction, whether through alignment or affiliation. In this chapter, we will further define *capital*, highlight the various capital procurement options available to parties who wish to align or affiliate, discuss how each source of capital typically is used in each of the affiliation models as outlined in the previous chapters and presented in Figure 16.1, below.

Also, we will highlight the relative cost associated with each form of capital as well as the implications of using each form of capital on investors. The use, source, risk, cost, and impact to ownership are factors to consider carefully when deploying capital.

As described in Chapter 4, limited integration models involve relationships among the relevant parties that stop short of significant long-term integration/affiliation. Moderate integration models attempt to address more ongoing and lengthier affiliations, though not permanent. Full integration involves high levels and prospectively longer-term or permanent forms of affiliation.

When considering capital in a broad sense as financial resources, the range of its sources is extensive and its procurement process can range from relatively simple to quite complex. To narrow the definition of capital here, we are focusing on economic capital, which can be categorized as financial or non-financial in nature and can be sourced internally or externally.

FINANCIAL CAPITAL

Financial capital is defined as the economic resource measured in terms of cash (or its equivalent) used or needed to fulfill a desired alignment

FIGURE 16.1. Alignment Models, Integration Level, and Typical Source(s) Capital

Affiliation Model	Integration Level	Source of Capital
Managed Care Networks	Limited	Internal - Cash
Recruitment/EPPM/PSM	Limited	Internal - Cash
Group (Legal-Only) Merger	Limited	Internal - Cash
Call Coverage Stipends	Limited	Internal - Cash
Medical Directorships	Limited	Internal - Cash
Service Line Management	Moderate	Internal - Cash
MSO/ISO	Moderate	Internal - Cash
Clinical Co-Management	Moderate	Internal - Cash
Equity Group Assimilation	Moderate	Internal - Cash
Joint Ventures	Moderate	Internal - Cash / External - Debt and Equity / Non-Financial
ACO/CIN	Full	Internal - Cash / External - Debt
Employment "Lite"	Full	Internal - Cash
Employment	Full	Internal - Cash
Group (Legal and Operational) Merger	Full	External - Debt and Equity
Private Equity Affiliation	Full	External - Equity

or affiliation strategy. Financial capital can be sourced internally (i.e., cash-on-hand) or externally, where funds are sourced from the capital markets (i.e., debt financing or equity investors).

Internal Financial Capital

Internal financial capital is the cash an entity has on-hand that can be used to effectuate an affiliation. Myriad factors can affect the level of available cash an entity may have available to fund an affiliation or transaction. Although not an exhaustive list, considerations include the lifecycle stage of the company, the typical or standard level of equipment and other tangible asset investment needed for effective operations, and current debt service requirements, to highlight just a few.

Internal financial capital is used typically when the capital requirement is not significant. This aligns well within limited affiliation models and most moderate affiliation models (as outlined in Figure 16-1 and discussed in detail in Chapter 4). Within these types of affiliation models, except for joint ventures and larger, more capital-intensive integrations, capital most often is needed to help fund the associated professional fees (e.g., legal costs, fair market value opinions, due diligence) in connection with completing the affiliation strategy.

The key benefit of using internal capital is that it is the cheapest form of capital. Its use prevents dilution to equity holders, and no associated principal or interest payments would result from debt financing. Consequently, if internal financial capital is available and can be used toward the capital outlay needed to effectuate the affiliation, it should be considered as a primary choice for capital procurement.

External Financial Capital

External financial capital represents capital raised in the capital markets—that is, debt capital from financial institutions willing to lend or invest money or equity investors. A brief discussion of these two sources of external capital follows.

Debt Financing

Debt financing typically is sourced from financial institutions such as banks or the sellers themselves (i.e., seller-financed deals). As debt capital is *cheaper* than equity capital due to the recourse and scheduled return of investment, entities always seek to optimize their level of debt financing before going to the equity markets to find outside equity investors. With the deployment of external capital, risk for the entity increases as does the cost of the capital (e.g., interest payments). Lending sources will want to reduce their risk of repayment by seeking collateral.

When procuring debt capital from a financial institution, collateral is generally secured in connection with a loan; the borrower pays both scheduled principal and interest payments over the term of the loan. Although debt holders do not have ownership rights, their position in the capital structure is higher (i.e., their claim on assets is superior to equity holders) as they have recourse through the collateralized assets. The risk to investors is also considered lower when compared to equity capital, due to the regular return of capital through principal and interest payments.

As Figure 16.1 shows, debt financing is most often used in conjunction with the investment in technology needed to start an accountable care organization (ACO), clinically integrated network (CIN), or when it can be used in conjunction with equity financing as part of a joint venture or group merger.

Another form of debt capital is evident in seller-financed deals, which are affiliations in which the principal and interest payments are made directly to the seller over a specified deal term instead of going to a financial institution. This type of capital procurement is common when a physician practice purchases another physician practice. Like debt financing through a financial institution, the seller does not retain any ownership rights in the practice but does have a higher claim on the underlying assets until all principal and interest payments have been made.

Depending on the terms offered by financial institutions, this form of debt capital often can cost less while providing an opportunity for the buyer and seller to remain engaged post-transaction.

Equity Financing

Equity financing is the method of raising capital by selling new ownership interests in the subject entity to investors. Although there are multiple forms of equity investment, this discussion focuses on preferred and common equity, with the key differences being the associated rights attributable to each type.

Regardless of the kind of equity investment, equity capital almost always is the costliest form of capital procured in an affiliation. The higher cost associated with equity financing is synonymous with the higher return equity investors require based on their position in the capital hierarchy. Equity holders generally receive a distribution or dividend only after other required payments of the entity have been met.

This additional level of uncertainty has more risk than collateralized debt and, therefore, bears an increased cost to the entity seeking capital. Furthermore, equity investment can dilute the value of the ownership interests held by current owners of the practice. Each of these factors must be considered as part of the overall affiliation strategy when thinking about equity financing.

Preferred equity holders often realize a specified dividend. This dividend is guaranteed in the sense that before any distributions to common equity holders are made, the required dividend to preferred equity holders must be completed. In exchange for this dividend, however, preferred equity holders generally do not have the same ownership rights as common equity holders. Preferred equity holders typically are higher in the capital structure (i.e., they have a senior claim on assets over common equity should liquidation of the company occur) and thus have a lower cost of capital (or return required by investors) compared to common equity holders.

Common equity holders typically invest in anticipation of material business growth to earn a return on their base investment. This contrasts with preferred equity holders and debt financing, which has a built-in mechanism for the investor to receive a return on their investment in the form of dividends (preferred equity), payment of principal and interest (debt financing). Common equity is also lower in the capital structure (i.e., it often has the last claim on assets should liquidation occur) and, thus, is viewed with more risk. Because of the higher perceived risk, the required return to the investor is greater and the cost of that capital deployed by the entity is more expensive.

Although less applicable when considering affiliation strategies, current owners of a practice could invest additional capital in return for additional member units in the practice. This type of equity raise is more common if the practice wants to expand to a new site or purchase new equipment. As such, we have not explored this form of external equity capital further within this chapter.

When considering external equity capital, such as with private equity, the affiliation model often involves a platform practice, which is a sizeable well-managed practice. Although a detailed discussion is outside the scope of this book, it is important to note that private equity firms raise their capital from institutions and wealthy individuals and then invest that money to buy and sell businesses. These deals almost always consider a 100% equity purchase of the subject practice. Private equity investors also appear in the context of the purchase of specialty practices, as these practices often drive the ancillary revenue associated with other investments owned by the private equity firm.

Non-Financial Capital

Non-financial capital is defined as economic resources measured in terms of non-financial assets used or needed to fulfill a desired alignment or affiliation strategy. Non-financial assets include fixed assets (e.g., equipment) and intangible assets (e.g., tradename). Non-financial capital typically is internally sourced and includes assets owned and contributed as capital by one or more parties to an affiliation. As the assets are already owned, the associated cost of procuring this capital has already been incurred. Consequently, only the opportunity cost of using this form of capital in an affiliation must be considered. To help assess the opportunity cost, each party often performs a valuation of their assets to ensure that the consideration received for the contributed assets is consistent with fair market value.

Utilizing non-financial capital is a common capital procurement strategy associated with joint ventures where one or more parties contribute non-financial assets in lieu of cash or equity investment. For the parties to then retain or reach a desired equity split in the joint venture, internal financial capital (i.e., cash) or external financial capital (i.e., equity or debt) can be contributed to reaching the desired ownership in the newly formed joint venture.

OTHER CONSIDERATIONS

All affiliation models require some form of capital procurement, whether it is cash, debt, equity, or non-financial assets. Multiple sources of capital usually must be explored for larger or more complicated affiliations. Although it is essential to understand the cost of capital associated with all affiliation models, this exercise becomes more critical and complicated when multiple sources of capital are involved.

In these instances, it is advisable to have an expert run various cost of capital scenarios to gain a better understanding of the options as well as the future impact the concluded capital procurement strategy will have on the parties. Furthermore, in connection with external capital and non-financial capital, a valuation of the subject entity and/or contributed assets is often required for the successful implementation of the affiliation.

SUMMARY

In this chapter, we defined capital, highlighted the various capital procurement options available to the parties, discussed how each source of capital is typically used in each of the affiliation models, and highlighted the relative cost of each form of capital as well as the resulting implications from the use of capital on investors.

Because of the varying costs of capital and the impact each type of capital can have on investors on an ongoing basis, detailed analyses must be performed to understand the implications of capital procurement in every affiliation. Furthermore, depending on the type of affiliation model being considered as well as the capital that may exist internally, the procurement of capital can come from multiple sources and can range from simple to complex. In more complicated affiliations, it is common to engage third-party consultants to aid in the cost of capital analyses and/or the valuation of the subject entity/assets involved in the affiliation.

As with all aspects of affiliation models, the more informed you can be related to your capital procurement options, the smoother the affiliation process will be for all parties involved.

CHAPTER 17

Transaction Mechanics and Key Steps of the Deal Process

Throughout this book, we have detailed various transaction models that are common among healthcare services organizations in the current marketplace, as well as some critical considerations for leaders as they pursue such transactions.

In addition to understanding the various models and some of the characteristics associated with these types of transactions, leaders involved must have at least a basic understanding of some of the mechanics of the transactions.

Every transaction, just like every healthcare organization, has unique characteristics and nuanced circumstances; therefore, it is impossible to encapsulate every variable that may emerge throughout a particular deal process. Nevertheless, we will address some of the higher-level components of a transaction and outline some key steps of a deal process. This knowledge can help leaders develop a strategy that leads to completing an efficient transaction that returns quantifiable value to all stakeholders.

OVERVIEW OF THE DEAL PROCESS

No two transactions are alike, even those involving similar organizations, structures, and models. Nevertheless, there are similar steps, milestones, and procedures that leaders can follow when pursuing a transaction. These somewhat standardized processes can apply for all types of transactions, from major health system merger and acquisition deals to hospital-driven acquisitions of ancillary services entities to the sale of a physician practice to hospital-physician employment, and everything in between. Figure 17.1 illustrates some of the key steps.

FIGURE 17.1. Steps in the Deal Process

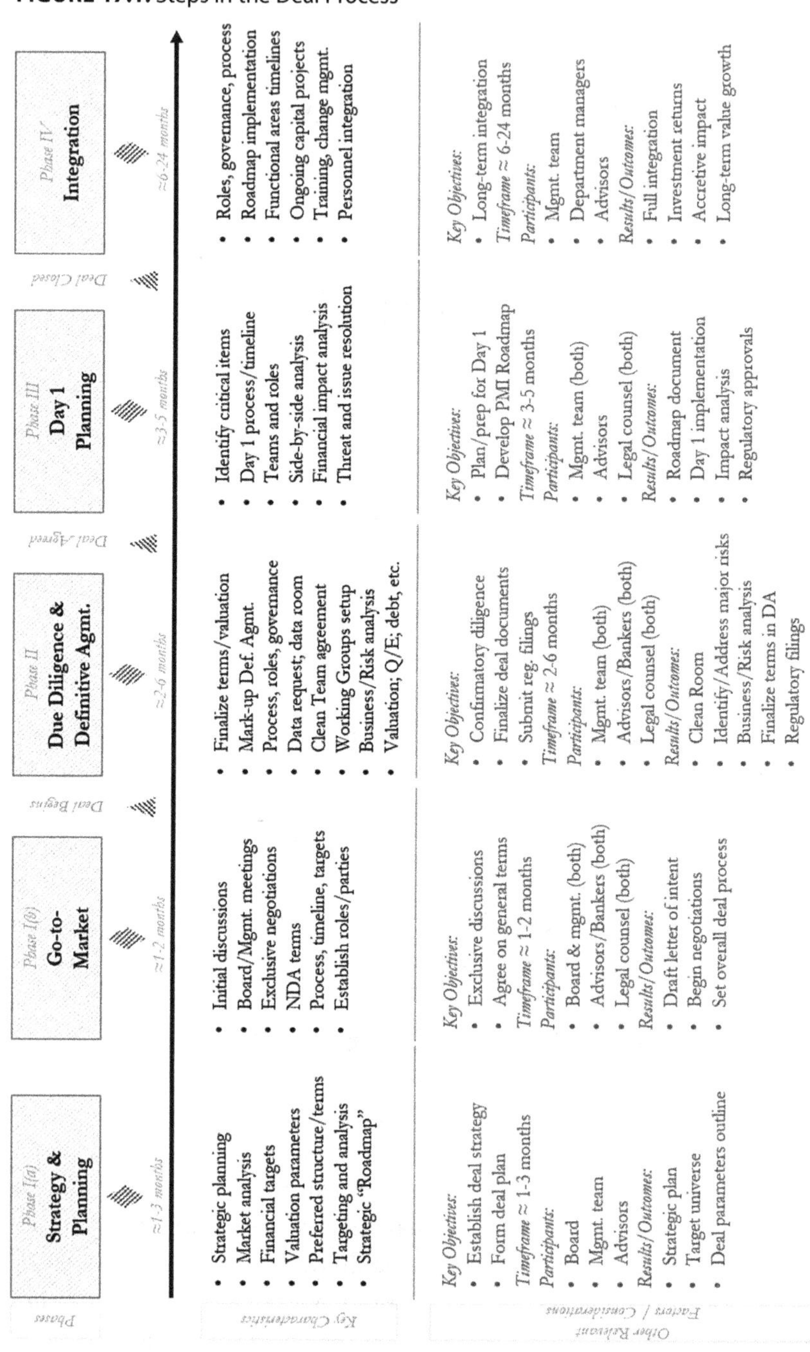

The information related to each step in the graphic and that we outline in this section is somewhat generic in that each transaction will dictate the specific elements, milestones, and timelines required. These steps and the related information are intended to present general elements and common characteristics.

With that understanding, let us address the typical vital components of healthcare transactions in further detail.

Phase I(a) – Strategy and Planning

Many deals seem to start with a representative from one party having a discussion—often a very casual or even unintentional conversation—with representatives from another party, which eventually culminates with the parties pursuing some type transaction. This scenario does not apply exclusively to small deals. Transactions involving major health systems in which the deal value is over $100 million can begin when the CEO of the buyer organization has dinner with a sub-set of the seller's shareholders. Here, the discussion developed with a comment that went something like, "Hey, we think you guys would fit well within our organization. What do you think about us buying you?"

This initial casual approach does not necessarily guarantee success or failure or results in a transaction. The point is that many deals begin more or less on a whim. While positive outcomes are not impossible in these scenarios, this approach is not always optimal, especially in the current marketplace of highly competitive transactions and challenging hurdles to make deals work in the long run.

We are not just referring to the idea that the definition of success is the lack of failure. Instead, making deals work is defining success by the achievement of long-term value for all stakeholders involved.

So, if we are pursuing the creation of long-term value for all stakeholders, it is safe to assume that should entail a significant amount of planning and analysis, likely with multiple rounds of discussion. Before an organization can map out these items, it will first need to define the objective, the parameters and constraints for pursuing that objective, and the desired outcomes the stakeholders wish to achieve. A critical element in all this is leadership; leaders will formulate and direct a vision. With the key individuals driving an initiative, they can dive into the other steps.

This strategy and planning phase essentially indicates that the organization has not necessarily arrived at the actual deal phase of the process. This stage is a preliminary initiative, but it is a vital part of the overall process because the leaders driving this initiative have an opportunity to set the objectives and targets and can set a tone for the overall process, which will increase the chances of a deal's success. Those leaders who are willing to invest the time and resources into diligently planning will achieve greater success over time through their various transactions.

Moreover, these organizations are almost always more dynamic and prepared when it comes to dealing with the inevitable challenges that are likely to emerge in any deal process—which results in reduced costs, enhanced risk mitigation, and shorter timelines.

Some critical components of a deal strategy include:

- Defining the strategic vision for the desired transaction (i.e., the rationale of the deal).
- Setting targets, parameters, and constraints.
- Conducting market analyses.
- Completing initial financial analyses (i.e., budgeting, capital constraints, etc.).
- Outlining optimal (or acceptable) structure and economic/non-economic terms.
- Formulating initial targeting list of buyers/sellers.
- Creating a roadmap for the transaction process.

This phase can incorporate many different elements and an organization can complete a number of steps at this point. That said, however, this phase is one that can also be scaled up or down, depending on the unique characteristics of a specific deal scenario.

For example, if a hospital is acquiring a three-physician primary care practice under a traditional employment model, it is safe to assume this may not require months (or even weeks) to create a detailed strategic plan. However, if a health system is considering a professional services agreement (PSA) with a 50-physician surgical specialty group that also entails the acquisition and/or joint venture equity purchase of ancillaries and the exchange of other assets, this requires diligent planning before taking those first steps. Likewise, if a physician practice of any size is considering selling to a private equity buyer resulting in up-front money and ongoing employment, which will permanently change how that entity works, then there may be only one opportunity to get things right. This transaction warrants a healthy degree of planning and intentional visioning.

Those prospects and initial selling points of a deal discussed casually over dinner may appear attractive and have a great deal of appeal on the surface. However, merely having a feeling that an idea makes sense is an entirely different thing compared to the intentional, proactive, and diligent consideration of what is optimal. In many healthcare transactions, the parties share that initial gut feeling that what they are talking about makes sense, but this conclusion is not always enough to achieve success. Therefore, we encourage leaders to devote the appropriate amount of time, resources, and attention to this strategy and planning phase.

Phase I(b) – Go-to-Market

While the *go-to-market* step could often be recognized as a phase of a deal process, it is the second component to the first phase because this step typically is something that occurs as a natural progression between the two parties.

Progressing from planning into the go-to-market phase, if successful, will allow us to reach our first significant milestone, which is essentially the launch point of the deal itself. As discussed earlier, this step is not something that should be underestimated or glazed over, because diligence in this portion of the process can ultimately determine success over failure or perhaps degrees of it.

The go-to-market phase is like a pre-deal step. The assumption that both or all of the parties agree to meet and explore potential affiliation. The details are yet to be defined. Nothing is binding except confidentiality terms. Executing the appropriate non-disclosure agreements (NDAs) is a key component of this phase.

As the parties come together, the high-level discussions about a potential affiliation begin. This introduction does not necessarily mean that these discussions must remain at a high level. Typically, this is more of a courting phase, where the talks most likely will be positive and forward-looking, with the real meat of negotiations to come later.

This stage is an excellent opportunity for the parties to establish ground rules or general parameters of the deal. Depending on the scenario, a buyer may be competing with other players for the opportunity to proceed in the pursuit of the seller. In this case, because the seller probably will need to evaluate different variables to decide in which direction to proceed, they likely will require specific information from interested parties.

These competitive scenarios, often referred to as bake-offs, typically are structured and eventually managed by an outside advisor, such as a consulting or mergers and acquisitions advisory firm. The seller, working with their advisor in this case, can direct the process in such a way that allows them to obtain the information needed for the key stakeholders to make an informed decision as to the optimal path.

As with all transaction scenarios, there are many elements in a situation like this that extend beyond the scope of this discussion. However, the main point here is that this phase of the deal process is an opportunity for the parties to come together and set the initial foundation for what will hopefully be a productive and successful transaction.

Some of the critical components of the go-to-market phase include:

- Engaging in initial deal discussions, typically at a board or management level.
- Identifying parties, including advisors, and outlining optimal process steps.
- Executing NDAs and other confidentiality provisions between all relevant parties.
- Outlining process timeline, milestones, roles, and other relevant parameters of the process.
- Mapping out next steps and action items necessary to proceed.

Like each step to completion, the timeline for this phase can vary and the nature of each deal will eventually dictate the range for scaling the timeline up or down. In competitive scenarios, these timelines often can extend due to the number of moving parts that such cases entail. The other side of that equation, however, is that these types of processes often are well organized and effectively managed, in addition to the clear communication of expectations, all of which often are well worth the compromise of the process taking longer.

Also, most deals involving larger organizations and as a result, relatively high economic terms (i.e., valuations) will typically require more time in this stage. There will often be more to discuss, in addition to more regulatory compliance requirements that usually are not involved in smaller-scale transactions.

Nevertheless, smaller transactions are not always quicker or more straightforward to proceed through the go-to-market phase. Ironically, the relatively small deals seem to drag the most in what gradually feels like a never-ending discussion phase. A transaction can stagnate in this form of affiliation purgatory.

One of the best ways to prevent this standstill or push through a stagnation period is to revisit the items outlined in Phase I. The more organizations invest in the planning stages, the more likely they are to push through the hurdles. If it becomes apparent the targets cannot be achieved, they are quick to move on entirely, which is sometimes the best option. Nevertheless, allowing things to drag on for extended periods without any meaningful progress is rarely productive for any of the parties involved.

Phase II – Due Diligence and Transaction Agreements

Now that we have progressed through the planning stage and laid the groundwork through the initial courting stage, we finally are ready to proceed with what most people assume is the first stage of a transaction process. When we see a potential deal begin from that casual discussion over dinner, the parties often agree that it is time to dive into due diligence and formulate the necessary affiliation agreements. However, as we have continued to point out, this step will almost always be far more successful if the parties have invested adequate time and resources into those first stages. If so, we can expect this stage to run more smoothly in one direction or another, which is to say the parties can ultimately reach that go/no-go milestone without unnecessary hair-pulling or chess matches that can negatively slow the process or create major roadblocks.

This phase requires the most work in terms of heavy lifting. The consultants, advisors, and legal counsel must dominate to ensure all the necessary items are addressed and nothing slips through the cracks. Allowing the outside advisors to drive this critical stage can also help move forward in a positive manner because they can proceed without emotions and relationship dynamics.

It is essential to let the outside advisors finalize the items in this phase objectively. Allowing them to "be the bad guys" means that when all is said and done, the consultants, lawyers, and the rest will go on their way to their other clients or the next deal. Then, it is the affiliating organizations and their respective stakeholders who must make this new venture work together.

If a deal falls through, the organizations involved still must go on with their respective businesses in their respective markets where long-term stability is always a factor. This is not the time to let emotions or egos impede achieving the bigger picture of success.

Finally, it is the outside advisors—consultants, attorneys, bankers, et al.—who deal with these transactions daily and who have the experience, insight, and skillsets to address the needs that will arise in this stage of the process. If they are representing your organization's interests, which they should be, then letting them do what they are engaged to do will be the optimal decision for all parties.

Some of the critical components of this phase include:

- Collect data and documentation necessary for due diligence.
- Set up appropriate tools for exchanging information (e.g., data site, Clean Room, etc.).
- Establish working groups that include appropriate individuals from all parties.
- Conduct various business, compliance, operational, and risk analyses .
- Complete valuation analyses, quality of earnings (Q/E), balance sheet analyses, etc.
- Set groundwork for integration planning.
- Draft appropriate affiliation agreement documents (letter of intent, definitive agreement, etc.).

The timeline for the due diligence and affiliation agreements phase is longer than for the other aspects of the deal process because of the amount of work that is typically involved in this stage, even for relatively smaller transactions. Due to the high degree of regulatory compliance requirements for healthcare services organizations, there typically will be more items to address in due diligence.

With that in mind, recognize that even a general estimate of two to six months for completing due diligence is likely on the aggressive schedule. Again, the larger the deal is in terms of economic scale and/or the size of organizations involved, the more burdensome the due diligence process likely will be.

A discussion of transaction due diligence includes two key points of emphasis.

First, the parties must acknowledge that due diligence should not be in only one direction; due diligence should entail the buyer not just evaluating the seller, but should also incorporate reverse due diligence. Although this review may not be as extensive as the primary due diligence, a seller should take advantage of the opportunity to confirm and validate the decision to pursue a particular path through reverse due diligence.

Second, due diligence should not be treated as a checklist exercise in which the buyer looks under the hood of the seller to confirm there are no major nuclear threats that would warrant killing the deal. Far too many deals occur in which one of the parties—typically the buyer—soon after the closing discovers a growing list of problems that perhaps did not surface in the due diligence phase as "deal killers." These problems turned out to be major landmines that negatively impacted their expectations for success.

These situations require considerable remediation, which is why we emphasize the necessity for extensive due diligence as a part of integration planning before completing a deal. There are many variables to consider, but the bottom line is to approach due diligence as an opportunity to both identify problematic issues and begin laying the groundwork for post-merger integration and optimization. This initiative inevitably will increase the chances for success and likely shorten the timeline for achieving it as well.

Phase III – Day One Planning

The third phase of the deal process primarily builds on the concept of using due diligence as the foundation for integration planning. Objectively, this information provides the opportunity to look ahead and plan for the future, specifically in terms of resolving challenge areas and optimizing opportunities to capitalize on key areas of value.

Many transactions involving healthcare services organizations enter a period of limbo, which we describe as "deal purgatory." Unlike the feeling of stagnation that the parties can manage and control, this stage is agonizing, uncontrollable, and unavoidable. This is the period during which legal counsel addresses the appropriate regulatory documentation, filing, and approval processes required for transactions relating to certain types of healthcare entities. These requirements and the accompanying procedures vary based on the size of the organizations, the scale and structure of the deal, and various local, state, and federal regulatory and/or legal guidelines. Many healthcare transactions are delayed because although the deal is set, the final agreements cannot be sealed until specific items are addressed, resolved, and in some cases, approved by the appropriate authorities.

Although the deal seems to stall at this point, waiting for the final items to be addressed, this period offers an opportunity for the parties to keep working toward the integration objectives, even if only to continue the integration *planning*. In some cases, this can cause the legal counsel some anxiety in that they do not want anything to negatively influence the outcome of those regulatory approval procedures, and rightfully so.

Likewise, the parties of the transaction—the buyer and seller—may be reticent to go too far down this path. If for some reason the deal was derailed they would not only have wasted their efforts, they potentially would have exchanged sensitive information that could negatively impact the organizations after the termination of the process.

These concerns are valid, and the parties should make an effort to incorporate the relevant variables and constraints in their respective situations. Nevertheless, the emphasis here is Day One planning, which refers to a specific effort of planning for integration, continuing from due diligence, which begins when the initiative takes effect. This is a perfect opportunity to refine the focus, drilling down specifically into planning for the Day One "go-live" event that will occur with the execution of the final agreements.

Now, the heavy lifting of the transaction itself is over. After the regulatory procedures are completed and the necessary approvals are obtained, the only remaining activity is to sign on the dotted line. Once that happens, the deal is complete and the previously separate parties are now one. The stakeholders must make this transaction work.

The two leaders from these organizations may find themselves in a couple of scenarios. In one case, the stakeholders could complete the final documents and then speculate, "Now what?" The alternative has the stakeholders completing the formal agreements and being ready to say, "Flip the switch!"

The first scenario suggests that after all the time and effort expended in getting the deal done, the parties must figure how they will make this whole venture work. The deal advisors and attorneys have concluded their work; thus, unless they have a plan and outside advisors engaged and mobilized to implement the plan, the organization will fight an uphill battle or, at best, work against a more challenging clock.

However, if the stakeholders used every opportunity to conduct the necessary planning and mobilize the appropriate resources, including both internal working groups and outside advisors, then at go-live, the stakeholders will be positioned to achieve their targeted objectives.

Critical components of this phase include:

- Identify areas using the "red/yellow/green" assessment.
- Develop the integration roadmap, which will start with Day One.
- Formulate a unique Day One integration plan, which entails immediate implementation.
- Establish teams, roles, reporting structures, governance, documentation protocols, etc.
- Develop a plan for issue resolution as well as programs for immediate value capture.
- Construct appropriate budgets, capital planning, financial projections, and more.

Having the Day One components in place should increase the likelihood for the parties to be able to "flip a switch" and begin integration. That first day is the most critical. Although it is unlikely that a major Y2K-like event will occur the day after a deal is done, the goal is to prevent the deal from experiencing adverse effects and maximize the opportunities for growth and value as soon as possible.

Phase IV – Post-Merger Integration

The last stage of the integration process, which ironically is the part most likely neglected, is the most significant factor in determining the long-term success of a transaction. It is also the portion of a deal that requires a separate discussion, which would fill another book. Nevertheless, it is essential to address integration and the role of integration within the overall transaction process here.

It is no mystery that, without effective integration, any efforts from the previous stages will, in the end, be for naught. Integration is not just tricky, though it can seem enigmatic. Getting a deal done is challenging; making it work is an entirely different level of complexity that entails variables and challenges that exceed anything likely to emerge in the deal process. Consequently, if an organization misses this piece, then all the positive interactions, good gut feelings, detailed analyses, and compelling intentions will mean nothing. Moreover, without effective integration, the organizations and the stakeholders involved will be left with major problems, including financial, operational, and perhaps legal.

The high-level keys to success in this stage entail comprehensive and diligent planning, the recruitment and mobilization of quality leadership, and the allocation of resources required to implement the optimal plan. Limited as to the depth of integration we can address in this material, we emphasize some of the important components in this stage:

- Implement the integration roadmap.
- Initiate change management and process improvement measures.
- Conduct training and other measures for the integration of personnel.
- Manage ongoing key performance indicators (KPIs) and integration milestones.
- Progress through appropriate phases of integration.

The scale of integration will always vary depending on the nature of each individual transaction; however, two fundamental tenants should be understood and embraced when it comes to integration. First, no matter the size, scale, or structure of a deal, some form of integration must occur. Second, integration does not happen without considerable planning, organization, and structure driving it. Integration cannot be felt-out-along-the-way. Success relies on a definitive plan that serves as the overall guide for working through the integration process.

A football team must be dynamic and flexible, able to make adjustments as needed throughout the course of a game or season. The team does not throw out the playbook every time a roadblock emerges. Similarly, the stakeholders involved in post-transaction integration must maintain a considerable degree of flexibility; however, if the playbook is designed appropriately before the process begins, the chances of success increase significantly.

SUMMARY

This chapter covers a relatively large amount of information, and considering the breadth of variables and factors that inevitably arise throughout a transaction process, barely scratches the surface. As we stressed often, no two deals are the same, and every transaction will have unique characteristics. Some deals have greater challenges than others; some seem to proceed without major hiccups despite the level of planning that was involved.

The principles covered in this chapter are somewhat generic and high-level, yet, they are helpful—and sometimes critical—when confronting the issue of not just completing a deal process, but completing it at a maximum level of optimization to produce long-term value far beyond the close of the deal.

CHAPTER 18

What Lies Ahead?

Healthcare in America is an ongoing discussion across the nation, for individuals, corporate executives, and politicians. Many unanswered questions remain concerning the future of affiliation transactions between healthcare entities. In this book, we have provided insights on various strategies and structures of affiliation as a reflection of the current healthcare "universe." It is essential to understand, appreciate, and consider the fundamental drivers of affiliation to prepare for the future. Payment and reimbursement structures are critical elements that drive affiliation transactions.

One answer to what lies ahead in alignment/affiliation transactions may be that the status quo continues whereby providers are compensated for the amount of work (volume) they do. Value-based reimbursement is discussed often and seems to be the trend of the future; however, it has not yet had a significant impact. Thus, if we are to continue under the same system, most providers will remain responsive to their volume of services with the incorporation of some consideration for quality in the corresponding reimbursement. Multiple payers are present in the market, including commercial and governmental, and they continue to talk about quality/value-based reimbursement while they pay mostly on volume.

Another debated trend for the future is the adoption of a single-payer system, although any such system likely will include an element of private insurance/risk support. We are concerned about the cost of healthcare and how best to manage it with our current and future systems of delivery and reimbursement. Indeed, the cost of a single-payer system is an enormous part of that debate. Some tout that single-payer systems entail a lower per-capita expenditure in other industrialized countries, yet many experts believe quite the opposite.

Unquestionably, under a single-payer system, government's (mostly federal) involvement causes costs to increase significantly. For example, Kenneth Thorp, Ph.D., Emory University professor of health policy, concludes that under a single-payer system pushed by many politicians these days, federal expenditures would increase by almost $25 trillion over a 10-year period.[1] Further, Charles Blahous, a senior research strategist at the Mercatus Center at George Mason University, estimates that such a plan would increase federal expenditures by $32.6 trillion during its first 10 years of implementation.[2]

Thus, from a cost perspective, all indications are that our current system, while far from perfect, would be better than a single-payer structure.

FEASIBLE OPTIONS FOR REIMBURSEMENT MODELS

One possible option for payment is to develop a hybrid system by combining fee-for-service and fee-for-value. Would some form of quality-based reimbursement that also entails ongoing fee-for-service reimbursement be best? Many have suggested that such a model would be too minor a change when we desperately need a more value-based reimbursement mindset. Others say that value-based reimbursement will be impossible to administer, much less quantify, on a major scale. The solution to date is to have some combination of fee-for-service that inclines more toward fee-for-volume.

Regardless of the reimbursement system in the United States over the next 10 to 20 years, providers and other healthcare entities must continue to work collaboratively toward achieving the best possible delivery model at the most efficient cost. It also must ensure that it compensates providers appropriately. Keeping these "balls in the air" and upholding them daily is incredibly challenging. Our healthcare system and its future, however, depend on achieving such standards.

Therefore, what drives alignment and affiliation models in the future will be the same issues that have propelled them in the past.

Drivers and Challenges of Affiliation/Alignment

We have identified 10 significant affiliation drivers (below) that apply regardless of the payer reimbursement system. A possible exception would be a single-payer system that would limit capitalism and free enterprise—the basis of many of the drivers listed.

1. **Quality of care.** The primary factor in affiliation model assimilation is delivering high-quality patient care. Practitioners are concerned about treating the patient for the most part, regardless of cost and economic ramifications.
2. **Management proficiency.** Managing any healthcare service entity is a daunting task, especially for providers who are less trained in practice management and are more familiar with the clinical services' delivery and care for patients. Managing a healthcare enterprise proficiently does not come easily; it takes a lot of experience and ability to address the issues that are day-to-day and longer-termed. For example, in a physician practice, the problems of adhering to regulations, ensuring proper coding and documentation, staying on the cutting-edge of revenue cycle recognition, and running the business day-to-day are incredibly challenging tasks that require highly trained and skilled professionals. These skills are expensive and drive the cost of private healthcare management upward. Therefore, the need to work collaboratively in affiliated models to achieve (afford) such levels of professionalism and proficiency in management is real and a plausible expectation.
3. **Recruitment and retention.** Procuring and maintaining an adequate supply of all types of providers, especially physicians, is demanding, and for the most part, the demand outweighs the supply. Though the demand and supply vary by locale, in the current healthcare delivery model, the entity must be able to recruit and then retain high-quality professionals in all areas of clinical services. The capacity to maintain a solid base of clinicians to ensure both quality and proficiency is essential, regardless of the system of delivery going forward. However, the responsibility for recruitment and retention may vary depending on the affiliation model.
4. **Provider compensation.** Highly trained and highly proficient clinicians (i.e., nurses, APPs, physicians, etc.) warrant a market-based compensation. Thus, as addressed in discussions of the various affiliation models, the providers' "employer" must arrange for market compensation. Even though many of the affiliation structures and models encompass incentives tied to quality and productivity, the compensation must be competi-

tive in the marketplace. Many believe that hospitals are the best entities to employ physicians and related providers, as they can best afford the costs. Though this view is debatable, affiliation models are often driven toward the ability of hospitals/health systems to meet provider compensation demands.

5. **Entity performance return on investment.** Fiscal viability is required of all healthcare service entities, even those that are not-for-profit, tax-exempt organizations. For-profit entities require a return on investment for their owner shareholders, which is among the considerations when exploring the affiliation model possibilities. Entity performance and return on investment should not be neglected or disapproved, even for a not-for-profit healthcare system, though it should not be the top priority. At the top of the list of important measures is rendering high-quality patient care. Nonetheless, fiscal performance is a driver of affiliation models.
6. **Technology and data.** The U.S. healthcare industry has been slow to develop technology and information assimilation, focusing more on the organization's financial performance rather than quality. Increasingly, healthcare is emerging as a technology data-driven industry, and rightfully so. However, technology initiatives are expensive and require significant investment to implement. Therefore, the ability to afford higher levels of technology and information exchange has prompted affiliation among all parties. Likewise, clinical technological advances are best made in collaboration with various provider and investor entities. The capacity to join in technological initiatives will continue to be a significant driver of affiliation models.
7. **Artificial intelligence and scientific advancement.** Similar to the need for technological development will be the demand for research and scientific progress to deliver more efficient and higher quality outcomes. Academic institutions can perform research and are equipped with the proper scientific and technological advances to drive value. The improvements in various areas of disease management and care, including cancer care, heart disease, and other specialties, are evidence of progress. Interested parties, including benevolent and academic institu-

tions and other providers, working together to complete the tasks of technological advances in clinical care, have proven beneficial.

8. **Academic mission.** We must commit to academic excellence to have proficient healthcare clinicians. This mission requires significant investment, collaborating with other providers and including physicians and health systems. Training the next generation of healthcare providers is a primary mission and objective of our healthcare industry today. Working together, collaboratively and through affiliations, will continue to be both an expectation and a requirement.
9. **Providing care for all.** We must extend benevolent care for all, regardless of background and the patient's ability to pay. Compassionate care encompasses many areas of responsibility and has political, social, and economic ramifications. Our country and healthcare system operate on the premise that no patient is denied care. We realize there are variations, depending on the institution and the providers rendering the care; nevertheless, safety nets are in place to ensure that care is provided to all our citizens, and even many non-citizens of the United States. Joining forces in affiliated models is and will continue as a major way to address such needs.
10. **Reimbursement means and overall delivery system.** As emphasized throughout the book, the ability to realize a return on investment starts (and some would argue stops) with the reimbursement structure. This emanates from both the government and private insurers and even to some extent from payments from the patients themselves. Collaboration and affiliation models will continue to be driven largely by this structure.

Driving Value in Healthcare Through Collaboration

How do we continue to promote and realize *real* value in the healthcare delivery system—both today and in the future—relative to collaborative initiatives? It is incumbent upon all of us in healthcare to keep our collective "eyes on this "ball."

We speak a lot about value-based payment systems and high-quality care and how to maintain them. To connect those dots, we talk about how the providers who deliver quality and efficiency in patient care should receive subsequent financial rewards. While the system is in a continual state of flux and fee-for-value versus fee-for-volume reimbursement is undefined, we still should strive to address these fundamental requirements within our healthcare delivery system for now and the future.

Following are some action steps to take and various forms of alignment/affiliation that are appropriate.

1. **Clinical alignment.** Health plans and providers must continue to work closely to align clinically. Achieving the best evidence-based treatment plans and disease management protocols is vital. Tying these together with appropriate reimbursement is equally important. Stakeholders today are taking a broader, more expanded view of clinical alignment. Coordination of care is not just a buzz term, it is a reality. It works. Decision making across continuums is critical. The effective system must be data-driven with tight integration that considers all the various factors, including some social determinates of best care.

   We applaud many health plans that are taking the lead on care management for complex disease management programs. This approach has delivered better cost controls, higher levels of patient satisfaction, and improved quality outcomes. Continuing this process will be essential as we move into the next decades.
2. **Economic alignment.** We speak a lot about this and indeed, it is justified. But there must be a bending of the cost curve and recognition of how costs of services affect the overall reimbursement structure and revenue "pie." Bundled payments for episodes of care are an example of how these matters could be realized going forward. Payers and providers sharing accountability for addressing chronic illnesses and for collaborative reimbursement make sense, and it works. It provides the necessary incentives to focus more globally on outcomes. Greater collaboration between payers and providers is the priority right now.
3. **Administrative alignment.** Healthcare is complicated, particularly the administrative management, accounting in general, and management oversight of the various healthcare entities. Merging providers, such as physicians, with proper administra-

tive management is sometimes like mixing oil with water—it is a challenge. The providers, all with a scientific background and expertise, are not always aligned with appropriate management and administrative protocols. Nonetheless, it is essential for success to have administrative alignment between payers, providers, and other healthcare entities, along with robust technology solution platforms. Providers must invest in a proper infrastructure with experience in administration to drive measurable and sustainable improvement to attain the proper results.

Key Considerations Relative to "What's Next"

Given the "moving parts" we have discussed, and our review in previous chapters, and now summarizing our key topic—that is, ways to affiliate and work collaboratively among healthcare providers and entities—here are the major takeaways. These guidelines apply to providers and all other healthcare service entities within our current system of care.

1. **Develop a strategic plan for the future.** A strategic plan serves as a vital guidebook or blueprint—it is not optional. Taking the time to invest in strategies for the future is the top priority, beyond anything else right now. It requires concerted thought, looking into the crystal ball to determine the future. The strategic plan also helps to define core values and cultures and how to address the inevitable challenges of today and tomorrow. The strategic plan will not be stagnant. It will not be perfect. It will be dynamic. It mirrors our healthcare industry and, therefore, the strategic planning process should never end.

   Some institutions and entities may be able to complete a strategic plan internally with the proper resources and expertise. Many entities require outside assistance, expertise from business advisors (even clinical advisors) to navigate the maze of considerations. Fundamentally, a strategic plan must always be front and center, updated, and stratified into key areas of importance and priorities.
2. **Maintain flexibility as to structures, affiliations, and overall alignment.** Whether it is a health system, private equity firm, physician practice, imaging or ambulatory surgery center, or

myriad other healthcare-related entities, it should share the mindset of flexibility. There is no permanent exclusive structure of affiliation or strategic plan initiative. Everything should be open to flexibility and plausibility, which can be a daunting yet invigorating aspect. Keeping an open mind to various models, areas of collaboration, and overall structure—both economically and practically—is obligatory.

3. **Consider a pluralistic approach to affiliation.** Similar yet more specific than the prior point, we emphasize the need for openness and willingness to consider various affiliation models. We have discussed numerous examples, devoting an entire chapter to some versions, believing each deserves consideration. Though not every approach is applicable, healthcare entities should understand their options and keep a mind open to the possible application of more than just one or two models.
4. **Respond to the marketplace.** Our healthcare industry is dynamic and evolutionary. With the formation of new entities, and the assimilation of new alignment consortiums, we see the development of new business plans that often reflect unique strategies that differ from anything done in the past. Local, regional, and national trends should be maintained with continued education and understanding. All point to the ability (albeit a necessity) for every healthcare entity to be responsive to market trends and realities. If they are not, continued viability (at least within their current structural make-up) is questionable.
5. **Listen to experts and educate every day.** While there are many so-called experts, the most reliable are those who have accrued knowledge through years of study and practical experience. We learn from history and from those who strive to understand how our healthcare system functions, today and in the future. It is essential to keep an open mind to these experts.
6. **Provide training and education at all levels of healthcare organizations.** The capacity to react to market trends and the various models of affiliation mainly will be attributable to understanding and training and how well an organization keeps-up with the trends. Fiscal viability should also be a priority.
7. **Communicate effectively.** Effective communication is easier said than done. Everyone is busy with tasks to complete. But

we must communicate well in all areas, whether with strategic planning, tactical issues, or day-to-day management and oversight. Interactions must be decisive, though concise and thorough, as inconsistent as the two may seem.

8. **Ask for help or understanding.** No individual or institution has all the answers. Everyone has legitimate questions and needs for clarification. Therefore, it is appropriate to adopt the premise that no question is a bad question.
9. **Do the right thing.** Acting or behaving correctly, appropriately, or with the best intentions is easier to say than do in our healthcare delivery system, though we harp on this issue a lot. The goal is to treat people properly, with respect, regardless of the relationship. Doing so is a winning initiative.
10. **Understand that change is relentless.** There are many areas of change to watch in order to remain current with the times. For instance, consider this (non-exhaustive) list of terms and/or initiatives and the movement that is occurring in these areas:
    - Value-based reimbursement
    - Telehealth
    - Utilization of APPs
    - Government regulations and adherence
    - Anti-trust considerations
    - Care coordination
    - Care delivery models
    - Roles of health systems versus physicians
    - Technology and related care information systems

The list is infinite and changes daily. We must always be cognizant and responsive to these and other significant initiatives.

SUMMARY

So, what lies ahead? Only the future will tell. We trust we have considered relevant issues that they will help you navigate the challenges of our healthcare delivery system and appropriate affiliation models and their structures. While dynamic and ever-changing, the models of affiliation we have presented are viable and proven. Further, with the proper structuring, including economic consideration, they are legal and regulatory compliant. They provide opportunities to enhance our healthcare delivery system, regardless of the reimbursement model and/or ownership structure.

REFERENCES

1. Thorp KE. An Analysis of Senator Sanders Single-Payer Plan. Healthcare-Now.org. January 27, 2016. Available at https://www.healthcare-now.org/296831690-Kenneth-Thorpe-s-analysis-of-Bernie-Sanders-s-single-payer-proposal.pdf. Accessed September 5, 2019.
2. Blahous C. *The Costs of a National Single-Payer Healthcare System.* Mercatus Working Paper, Mercatus Center at George Mason University, Arlington, VA; July 2018. Available at https://www.mercatus.org/system/files/blahous-costs-medicare-mercatus-working-paper-v1_1.pdf. Accessed September 5, 2019.

CHAPTER 19

Post-Crisis Affiliation

As we wrap up this book, the COVID-19 pandemic has turned our country and our planet upside down. Healthcare in the United States and worldwide will never be the same. This upheaval applies to all aspects of clinical care, including the alternatives for affiliation.

Affiliation options for physicians, the theme of this book, will be significantly affected going forward. For example, the interest and corresponding reimbursement improvements for telehealth/telemedicine services have already had a major effect due to the pandemic crisis. Affiliation relationships and transactions will undergo serious changes due to the advancement of telehealth services.

Healthcare providers—from hospitals to physician clinics and other entities—are impacted by this crisis. Going forward, crisis management will be a major influencer of any healthcare organization's strategy for partnering/affiliating with other entities.

Patients have changed as well, specifically in their attitude toward healthcare providers—not only by accepting telehealth services but by being more cautious about the way they interact with other human beings and in how they work with their healthcare providers.

Although hospitals and physician groups will continue to consider transactional opportunities, the arrangements may look different, including the economic and non-economic ramifications. The many employed or contracted physicians who have been placed on furlough or experienced a salary reduction may now be reticent to continue to affiliate with hospitals. Due to state and federal directives, many hospitals ceased elective surgeries and curtailed non-essential procedures during the crisis to focus strictly on COVID-19 patients. As a result, hospitals and health systems have experienced significant financial depletion of their cash reserves. Post-pandemic, it is uncertain whether they will see an immediate economic improvement in their bottom lines. These factors will affect their attitude toward affiliation transactions.

It is safe to say that all providers, investors, and especially American consumers have suffered and endured losses through the recent pandemic events. In trying to pull out of the crisis, there are many unanswered questions that we will consider throughout this chapter.

PHYSICIAN–HOSPITAL ALIGNMENT

After any crisis of the nature and magnitude of COVID-19, a desire for more security and an unwillingness to continue going it alone may lead to a rush to affiliate. Physicians are examining whether they can survive in a private setting. Hospitals are searching for means to recoup the lost revenue and earnings, including the not-for-profit hospitals that must have a positive financial performance to maintain their existence.

The question begs: Will hospitals and physicians be equipped financially to complete transactional affiliation deals when the pandemic subsides? While most transactions may entail negligible up-front capital, hospitals' economic reserves have dwindled; therefore, structuring a transaction with physician groups will be more challenging.

As noted, countless physicians may decide they cannot operate independently and will seek an affiliation that serves as an island of security. Hospitals and health systems will be the most likely cohorts. However, will the transactions be of a similar structure and present the economic ramifications as those we examined in earlier chapters?

We believe these transactions will predominate the marketplace, but the arrangements will be more conservative economically, at least for a while. Some hospitals may defer transactions for 6 to 12 months until they can "get on their feet" financially to assume these additional responsibilities. Similarly, any deals done will likely come with more strings attached, especially regarding compensation that is strictly tied to both production and quality-based performance metrics, placing physicians' compensation at an elevated level of risk.

The demand for physician-hospital affiliation transactions will remain high—perhaps even higher than during the pre-COVID-19 pandemic era. However, the transactions will look different due to the economic issues and the ever-growing presence of telemedicine.

The following key features may emerge after the COVID-19 pandemic:

1. Physicians will have an enhanced level of interest in affiliation and alignment.

2. The interest from hospitals will be more selective and, potentially, the compensation they offer to physicians less economically attractive. Contract structures may change, making the provider more at-risk by tying a greater amount of the total targeted compensation to production and clinical outcomes.
3. Hospitals will be able to select from physician groups that they believe are most important strategically and tactically, and most clinically proficient. This factor will depend on the overall quantity of physicians within their service area.
4. While the interest in alignment transactions will increase, the transaction processes may move more slowly. Hospitals at this stage have higher priorities than affiliations. Further, some physicians in private practice may be reticent to align as they return to their normal progression and volume of services.
5. The volume of telehealth services will continue to increase, which will influence the transactional value and paradigm established within the physician–hospital affiliation relationship.

PHYSICIAN-TO-PHYSICIAN AFFILIATION

Will more group mergers arise out of the COVID-19 pandemic crisis? That question is valid but difficult to answer. Group mergers of single specialties are usually easier to accomplish than multispecialty deals. Multispecialty group mergers are more challenging in that they involve more issues and areas of resolution. They often require an extended period to complete; therefore, post-pandemic, the first wave of affiliations will likely center on single-specialty group mergers. These affiliations could be under the banner of a clinically integrated organization (CIO) or some other loosely formed alliance, even if it is a merged entity that uses a single-provider number.

The challenges of merging will likely increase as the pandemic crisis wanes and given the economic hurdles, resolving issues may be more difficult than in the past. Increased capital is typically not a derivative of group mergers other than some cost economies of scale. Usually, increased cash flow is realized later as opposed to the nearer-term. Other reasons groups merge, such as the ability to project "strength in numbers" in payer contracting, vendor contracting, information technology (IT) aggregation, hospital relationships, and the ability to negotiate limited alignment transactions, will all be in play. Whether these factors will be sufficient in compelling physicians to pursue mergers is unknown.

Physician-to-physician affiliation post-pandemic may assume the following characteristics:

1. Multispecialty group mergers, while always a difficult challenge, likely will not be at the forefront.
2. Single-specialty mergers may create interest as an alternative, especially if hospital integration is not probable.
3. The reasons for merging will continue beyond the pandemic crisis, although mergers of all types of groups will be limited. Instead, providers will focus on more pressing financial needs and other concerns.
4. To the extent mergers are of interest, they likely will form as "legal-only" structures where operational combinations may be limited and/or deferred.
5. Many physician groups will seek a private equity investor in lieu of or in addition to group mergers.

PHYSICIAN–INVESTOR AFFILIATION

The physician–investor affiliation relates primarily to private equity (PE) firms investing in physician practices. Post-COVID-19 pandemic, investors' initial emphasis may be to address their existing investments rather than consider new deals. With 2020 earnings being considerably lower, there likely will be a period when additional rebounding of existing working relationships/investments is required. Moreover, this will give physician groups that might have otherwise been interested in a PE transaction more time to rebound.

Typically, multiples of EBITDA (earnings before income taxes, depreciation, and amortization) are the standards for the valuation of such transactions. Nowadays, the EBITDA has changed to an "EBITDAC," with the "C" standing for "COVID-19." The result is a reduction in earnings due to the pandemic crisis. Therefore, any deals considered post-pandemic, perhaps even for the first 12 to 24 months, will have the COVID-19 cloud over its structure, meaning that the EBITDAC will lower earnings and possibly the multiples on those earnings.

Whether this matter is a legitimate consideration is debatable. We believe it will be a serious component of future negotiations, at least for the next 12 to 24 months. Other industries, however, will not likely rebound as quickly as healthcare, and the market may actually improve sooner for PE-related transactions. Additionally, private equity may require groups to retain a higher ownership percentage, although still a minority interest, looking for a better valuation for all investors, including the physicians, within the "second bite of the apple" (i.e., subsequent sale).

From a physician-to-private-equity-investor standpoint, the following key areas are included in our post-COVID-19 forecast:

1. Private equity deals may be deferred for a short period as PE firms address the issues of existing investments post-COVID-19 pandemic.
2. Private equity firms will be a significant presence in the healthcare market—perhaps with a greater footprint there than in any other industry.
3. PE firms will be more selective, able to align with the "best" groups and consortiums because they will have an abundance of options.
4. Physician groups and related healthcare entity sellers to private equity investors may have to retain greater equity (a more considerable minority interest) and be willing to accept lower multiples on EBITDAC.
5. In general, private equity organizations will be aggressive, but selective, and still subscribe to significant ROI, imposing more stress on the physicians to perform post-transaction.
6. Physician groups will be challenged to convince their partners to pursue a PE transaction. Compensation reductions that result from PE deals will not be well-received, given the significant loss of income in 2020 due to the COVID-19 pandemic.

VALUATION AND COMPENSATION RAMIFICATIONS

As discussed previously, though indirectly, the critical areas of consideration will be historical and future projected profits (i.e., EBITDAC) upon which valuations will be based, and the post-transaction compensation parameters. These include the pay reduction not only to create up-front earnings but to mitigate COVID-19 pandemic losses. The latter works both ways as physicians are looking for opportunities to improve their compensation. At the same time, PE firms, hospitals, and other practice purchasers do not want to lose as much money from employing physicians, given the economic stresses created by the pandemic.

Valuation approaches will continue to focus on the market and income methodologies but, again, will be based on more conservative (lower) historical earnings, plus even more conservative projections for the future. Valuation firms must be savvy, on top of the latest trends in assigning multiples, and not reliant on industry benchmark surveys that have not had time to react and respond to the COVID-19 pandemic effects on compensation and productivity. In other words, the past trends and precedents may not be best applied, at least initially, until the effects of COVID-19 are documented.

Independent appraisal firms will still be at the focal point of the transactions and, as noted above, should be up-to-date on the latest trends and resultant assumptions that form the foundation of valuations going forward. This will apply not only to the economic terms, but also their regulatory and legal ramifications.

Post-pandemic transaction physician compensation will likely be lower, at least on a guaranteed basis, with more at-risk measures assigned. The ability to realize a legitimate "lift" in compensation post-transaction (which has historically been the case in virtually all areas of affiliation discussed herein) will be less prevalent. For the first time, we will experience benchmark-sourced compensation rates that are lower than in previous years.

SUMMARY

Affiliation strategies will continue post-pandemic. The previous chapters of this book still apply, and our view is that the key tenets of those transactions will continue for the most part. The deals effected by the post-pandemic crisis will result in some delays, economic changes, and additional changes due to strategic priorities for physicians, health systems, and private investors. So, many questions are yet to be asked and answered as we experience this pandemic crisis and its aftereffects.

We do not have all the answers specific to healthcare and within the strata of affiliation transactions. The entire dynamic is new, different, and uncharted. Therefore, look for continual changes and a potential "reinvention of the wheel." The desire is to return to some form of normalcy while being mindful of the immense changes that will result from the pandemic.

www.ingramcontent.com/pod-product-compliance
Lightning Source LLC
Chambersburg PA
CBHW060554220326
41598CB00024B/3103

9780984831098